Alternative and Complementary Therapies for Children with Psychiatric Disorders, Part 1

Editors

DEBORAH R. SIMKIN
CHARLES W. POPPER

CHILD AND ADOLESCENT PSYCHIATRIC CLINICS OF NORTH AMERICA

www.childpsych.theclinics.com

Consulting Editor
HARSH K. TRIVEDI

July 2013 • Volume 22 • Number 3

ELSEVIER

1600 John F. Kennedy Boulevard ● Suite 1800 ● Philadelphia, Pennsylvania, 19103-2899

http://www.theclinics.com

CHILD AND ADOLESCENT PSYCHIATRIC CLINICS OF NORTH AMERICA Volume 22, Number 3
July 2013 ISSN 1056–4993, ISBN-13: 978-1-4557-7582-8

Editor: Joanne Husovski
Developmental Editor: Donald Mumford

Child and Adolescent Psychiatric Clinics of North America (ISSN 1056-4993) is published quarterly by Elsevier Inc., 360 Park Avenue South, New York, NY 10010-1710. Months of issue are January, April, July, and October. Business and Editorial Offices: 1600 John F. Kennedy Boulevard, Suite 1800, Philadelphia, PA 19103-2899. Periodicals postage paid at New York, NY and additional mailing offices. Subscription prices are $297.00 per year (US individuals), $471.00 per year (US institutions), $149.00 per year (US students), $343.00 per year (Canadian individuals), $567.00 per year (Canadian institutions), $189.00 per year (Canadian students), $408.00 per year (international individuals), $567.00 per year (international institutions), and $189.00 per year (international students). International air speed delivery is included in all *Clinics* subscription prices. All prices are subject to change without notice. **POSTMASTER:** Send address changes to *Child and Adolescent Psychiatric Clinics of North America*, Elsevier Health Sciences Division, Subscription Customer Service, 3251 Riverport Lane, Maryland Heights, MO 63043. **Customer Service: 1-800-654-2452 (U.S. and Canada); 314-447-8871 (outside U.S. and Canada). Fax: 314-447-8029. E-mail: JournalsCustomer Service-usa@elsevier.com (for print support) or journalsonlinesupport-usa@elsevier.com (for online support).**

Reprints. For copies of 100 or more of articles in this publication, please contact the Commercial Reprints Department, Elsevier Inc., 360 Park Avenue South, New York, New York 10010-1710 Tel.: (212) 633-3812; Fax: (212) 462-1935, e-mail: reprints@elsevier.com.

Child and Adolescent Psychiatric Clinics of North America is covered in *MEDLINE/PubMed (Index Medicus), ISI, SSCI, Research Alert, Social Search, Current Contents,* and *EMBASE/Excerpta Medica.*

Printed and bound by CPI Group (UK) Ltd, Croydon, CR0 4YY

Transferred to digital print 2013

Contributors

CONSULTING EDITOR

HARSH K. TRIVEDI, MD
Associate Professor of Psychiatry, Vanderbilt University School of Medicine; Executive Medical Director, Chief of Staff, Vanderbilt Psychiatric Hospital, Nashville, Tennessee

CONSULTING EDITOR EMERITUS

ANDRÉS MARTIN, MD, MPH

FOUNDING CONSULTING EDITOR

MELVIN LEWIS, MBBS, FRCPSYCH, DCH

EDITORS

DEBORAH R. SIMKIN, MD
Distinguished Fellow, American Academy of Child and Adolescent Psychiatry; Medical Director, Attention, Memory and Cognition Center, LLC, Destin, Florida

CHARLES W. POPPER, MD
Clinical Associate in Psychiatry, Child and Adolescent Psychiatry, McLean Hospital; Clinical Instructor in Psychiatry, Harvard Medical School, Belmont, Massachusetts

AUTHORS

RYAN B. ABBOTT, MD, JD, MTOM
Associate Professor, Southwestern Law School, Los Angeles, California

L. EUGENE ARNOLD, MEd, MD
Professor Emeritus of Psychiatry, Nisonger Center, Ohio State University, Columbus, Ohio

ANNE-CLAUDE BEDARD, PhD
Department of Psychiatry, The Mount Sinai School of Medicine, New York, New York

ANIL CHACKO, PhD
Department of Psychology, The Graduate School and University Center, Queens College, City University of New York (CUNY), Flushing, New York; Department of Psychiatry, The Mount Sinai School of Medicine; Department of Child and Adolescent Psychiatry, New York University School of Medicine, New York, New York

MICHAEL H. COHEN, JD, MBA, MFA
Attorney-at-Law, Principal, The Michael H. Cohen Law Group, Beverly Hills, California

EMMELINE EDWARDS, PhD
Director, Division of Extramural Research, National Center for Complementary and Alternative Medicine (NCCAM), National Institutes of Health, Bethesda, Maryland

NICOLE FEIRSEN, BA
Department of Psychology, The Graduate School and University Center, Queens College, City University of New York (CUNY), Flushing, New York

ROBERT L. HENDREN, DO
Director, Child and Adolescent Psychiatry, Professor and Vice Chair, Department of Psychiatry, University of California, San Francisco, San Francisco, California

ELIZABETH HURT, PhD
Postdoctoral Researcher, Nisonger Center, Ohio State University, Columbus, Ohio

NICHOLAS LOFTHOUSE, PhD
Assistant Professor of Clinical Psychiatry, Ohio State University, Columbus, Ohio

DAVID MARKS, PhD
Department of Child and Adolescent Psychiatry, New York University School of Medicine, New York, New York

DAVID MISCHOULON, MD, PhD
Associate Professor of Psychiatry, Director of Research, Depression Clinical and Research Program, Massachusetts General Hospital, Harvard Medical School, Boston, Massachusetts

SUZANNE R. NATBONY, JD
Attorney-at-Law, Of Counsel, The Michael H. Cohen Law Group, Beverly Hills, California

CHARLES W. POPPER, MD
Clinical Associate in Psychiatry, Child and Adolescent Psychiatry, McLean Hospital; Clinical Instructor in Psychiatry, Harvard Medical School, Belmont, Massachusetts

MARK RAPAPORT, MD
Professor and Chair, Department of Psychiatry and Behavioral Sciences, Emory University School of Medicine, Atlanta, Georgia

SCOTT SHANNON, MD, ABIHM
Assistant Clinical Professor, Department of Psychiatry, University of Colorado, Colorado; Wholeness Center, Fort Collins, Colorado

DEBORAH R. SIMKIN, MD
Distinguished Fellow, American Academy of Child and Adolescent Psychiatry; Medical Director, Attention, Memory and Cognition Center, LLC, Destin, Florida

BARBARA STUSSMAN, BA
Survey Statistician, National Center for Complementary and Alternative Medicine (NCCAM), National Institutes of Health, Bethesda, Maryland

JODI UDERMAN, BA
Department of Psychology, The Graduate School and University Center, Queens College, City University of New York (CUNY), Flushing, New York

WENDY WEBER, ND, PhD, MPH
Program Officer, Division of Extramural Research, National Center for Complementary and Alternative Medicine (NCCAM), National Institutes of Health, Bethesda, Maryland

Contents

> Complementary and alternative medicine (CAM) defies simple definition, because the distinction between CAM and conventional medicine is largely arbitrary and fluid. Despite inconclusive data on the efficacy and safety of many CAM treatments in child and adolescent psychiatry, there are enough data on certain treatments to provide guidance to clinicians and researchers. CAM treatments, as adjunctive therapy or monotherapy, can be clinically beneficial and sensible. The low stigma and cost-competitiveness of many CAM psychiatric treatments are highly attractive to children and parents. Physicians need to be knowledgeable about CAM treatments to provide clinically valid informed consent for some conventional treatments.

Section 1: Complementary and Alternative Treatments for Specific Disorders

> Dozens of complementary and alternative treatments have been advocated for attention-deficit/hyperactivity disorder. Some verge into standard treatment of specific cases. Most do not have conclusive evidence of effectiveness or safety for attention-deficit/hyperactivity disorder, but some have enough evidence and are safe, easy, cheap, and sensible enough that individual patient trials can be justified. There is a need to flesh out the evidence base, which could be done cost effectively for supplements or off-label agents that are amenable to placebo control.

> The therapeutic value of physical exercise, bright light therapy and dawn simulation, and several pharmacologic treatments, including hypericum (St. John's wort), S-adenosylmethionine, and 5-hydroxytryptophan, are reviewed, with a focus on their use for treating major depressive disorder in children and adolescents and also for alleviating depressed mood in the general (nonclinical) population of youth. For each treatment discussed, all published randomized, double-blind, placebo-controlled trials are summarized, along with some additional selected studies. Nutritional psychopharmacology and several other approaches to treating depression will be presented in an upcoming volume in the *Child and Adolescent Psychiatric Clinics of North America*.

Emmeline Edwards, David Mischoulon, Mark Rapaport, Barbara Stussman, and Wendy Weber

Complementary and integrative strategies are widely used by families with children who have mental health diagnoses. The therapies used by these children include herbs, dietary supplements, massage, acupuncture, meditation, and naturopathy. The literature on efficacy of complementary and alternative approaches is of limited value, and studies are needed to test efficacy and safety. Interpretation of complementary and integrative health care studies for symptomatic management of mental health conditions is hampered by study design and methodological limitations. Well-designed, adequately powered, and suitably controlled clinical trials on promising complementary and integrative modalities are needed for children and adolescents with psychiatric conditions.

CHILD AND ADOLESCENT PSYCHIATRIC CLINICS

RELATED INTEREST

Complementary Therapies in Medicine August 2011 (Vol. 19, No. 4)
Complementary Medicines (Herbal and Nutritional Products) in the Treatment of Attention Deficit Hyperactivity Disorder (ADHD): A Systematic Review of the Evidence
Jerome Sarris, James Kean, Isaac Schweitzer, James Lake

AACAP Members: Please go to www.jaacap.org for information on access to the Child and Adolescent Psychiatric Clinics. *Resident* Members of AACAP: Special access information is available at www.childpsych.theclinics.com.

DOWNLOAD
Free App!

Review Articles
THE CLINICS

NOW AVAILABLE FOR YOUR iPhone and iPad

Preface

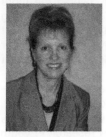 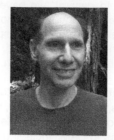

Deborah R. Simkin, MD   Charles W. Popper, MD
Editors

In deciding what topics to cover in this introduction to complementary and alternative medicine (CAM) treatments in child and adolescent psychiatry, we were primarily interested in focusing on treatments backed by useful research—data that allow us to evaluate the clinical value of these treatments for youth with psychiatric disorders. The CAM treatments covered here have been chosen because the available data in youth allow some inferences about their effects (positive or otherwise), because the limited data justify more research, or because of widespread public interest or common use of these treatments.

A huge variety of interventions were considered, but the scientific literature is too scant to support the meaningful discussion of most CAM treatments, especially in youth. We have found increasing activity and improving quality in CAM research in child and adolescent psychiatry, so the *Child and Adolescent Psychiatric Clinics of North America* have expanded their original plans and have allowed child and adolescent CAM psychiatry to be covered in 2 volumes. In these volumes, it will be clear that the data on many CAM treatments are often too limited to draw firm conclusions about their efficacy in youth, but are promising enough to offer helpful guidance to clinicians and researchers in child and adolescent psychiatry.

These 2 volumes are, by necessity, highly selective. CAM encompasses a vast range of types of treatments, systems of health care, and lifestyle philosophies. The selection of treatments discussed in these volumes tends toward the more conventional "near" side of CAM. We have not included alternative or non-Western systems of medicine. Acupuncture has gained a strong foothold in American medicine, even though its mechanism remains difficult to explain based on the Western traditions of anatomy and physiology. We have not included acupuncture in these volumes because we could not find any data regarding its use for psychiatric indications in youth (at least in the literature published in English). Chiropractic manipulation for physical conditions, although covered by health insurance companies, is supported by data, but the magnitude of its effects remains uncertain, and there are little data

Child Adolesc Psychiatric Clin N Am 22 (2013) ix–xi
http://dx.doi.org/10.1016/j.chc.2013.05.003
1056-4993/13/$ – see front matter © 2013 Published by Elsevier Inc.

childpsych.theclinics.com

on its value for treating psychiatric disorders and no data on child and adolescent psychiatric disorders. Prayer is sometimes included as a part of CAM, but again no controlled trials are available in youth. In general, we have not covered the more holisitic philosophies, which emphasize prevention, promotion of the self-healing functions of the body and mind, and the curative power of spirituality. At some point in the future, perhaps Ayurvedic medicine or Chinese herbs, or even homeopathy or energy therapies, might be systematically evaluated in child and adolescent psychiatry.

In this volume, we focus on CAM treatment approaches to several major psychiatric disorders in children and adolescents, specifically ADHD, mood disorders, autism, and certain learning disorders (reading disorder and disorder of written expression). We also deal with several general topics in CAM, including CAM research in youth (the issues and opportunities it presents), legal issues raised by prescribing CAM treatments in clinical practice and measures to minimize legal liability (including informed consent), and approaches to incorporating CAM into a clinical practice (and its implications for the professional development of a child and adolescent psychiatrist). While we are proud of all of our authors and their contributions, we are particularly honored that the lead author of the article on research is Dr Emmeline Edwards, the Director of the Division of Extramural Research at the National Center for Complementary and Alternative Medicine at the National Institutes of Health.

In the second volume on CAM in the *Child and Adolescent Psychiatric Clinics of North America*, which will be published in 2014, specific treatment techniques will be covered: neurofeedback (for ADHD, depression, anxiety, learning disorders, autism, brain injury, seizures, and addiction), mindfulness and meditation, music therapy (and music medicine), essential fatty acids, and micronutrients (vitamins and minerals) will be reviewed as treatments for psychiatric disorders in youth.

To provide consistency across articles, each CAM treatment has been ranked using the United States Preventive Services Task Force (USPSTF) system for grading the research evidence. Following the USPSTF guidelines, each CAM treatment has been assigned a grade for "Quality of Evidence" and a grade for "Strength of Clinical Recommendations" that can be made based on the evidence. This provides a uniform way of evaluating the relative value of available research on each CAM treatment. In addition to these evidence-based evaluations, we asked the authors to make personal recommendations based on the published literature in combination with their expert opinions based on their clinical experience. The treatment-oriented articles conclude with these 2 summary tables providing researchers with evidence-based evaluations and clinicians with clinically grounded evaluations of each CAM treatment.

We want to express our enormous gratitude to Elsevier for putting its innovative clinical focus on the topic of CAM treatments in child and adolescent psychiatry. We appreciate the support of series editor Dr Harsh Trivedi for granting 2 volumes to present this new material. And we especially wish to thank Joanne Husovski, our editor at Elsevier, with whom we worked very closely, for her incredible grace, knowledge, guidance, support, kindness in the face of the inevitable adversities, and invariable good cheer.

Deborah R. Simkin, MD
American Academy of Child and Adolescent Psychiatry
Attention, Memory and Cognition Center, LLC
4641 Gulfstarr Drive, Suite 106
Destin, FL 32541, USA

Charles W. Popper, MD*
Child and Adolescent Psychiatry
McLean Hospital and Harvard Medical School
Belmont, MA 02478, USA

E-mail addresses:
Deb62288@aol.com (D.R. Simkin)
Charles_Popper@harvard.edu (C.W. Popper)

*385 Concord Avenue, Suite 204
Belmont, MA 02478-3037, USA

Overview of Integrative Medicine in Child and Adolescent Psychiatry

Deborah R. Simkin, MD[a], Charles W. Popper, MD[b],*

KEYWORDS

- Complementary medicine • Alternative medicine • Integrative medicine
- Child psychiatry • Adolescent psychiatry • Stigma • Informed consent

KEY POINTS

- Complementary and alternative medicine (CAM) defies simple definition, because the distinction between CAM and conventional medicine is largely arbitrary and fluid.
- Despite the inconclusive data on the efficacy and safety of many CAM treatments in child and adolescent psychiatry, there are enough data on certain treatments to be useful to researchers and clinicians.
- The adjunctive use of (and sometimes monotherapy with) some CAM treatments may be clinically beneficial and sensible.
- Physicians need to be knowledgeable about CAM treatments to provide clinically valid informed consent for some conventional treatments.
- Physicians will find that venturing into CAM is often comparable to learning to use a novel conventional treatment.
- The low stigma and cost-competitiveness of certain CAM psychiatric treatments are highly attractive to children and parents.

The usual definitions of complementary and alternative medicine (CAM) imply a clear differentiation between CAM and conventional medicine, but the boundary between them is vague, arbitrary, fluid, and porous. Physical exercise as a treatment for serious medical diseases might have been considered unconventional and even radical 50 years ago, but exercise is now widely understood to benefit a broad range of medical conditions. There are innumerable examples of treatments that have converted from unconventional to established status. The introduction of the term integrative medicine implies that there is no need for this distinction between CAM and

[a] American Academy of Child and Adolescent Psychiatry, Attention, Memory and Cognition Center, LLC, 4641 Gulfstarr Drive, Suite 106, Destin, FL 32541, USA; [b] Child and Adolescent Psychiatry, McLean Hospital and Harvard Medical School, Belmont, MA 02478, USA
* Corresponding author. 385 Concord Avenue, Suite 204, Belmont, MA 02478-3037, USA.
E-mail address: Charles_Popper@harvard.edu

Child Adolesc Psychiatric Clin N Am 22 (2013) 375–380
http://dx.doi.org/10.1016/j.chc.2013.05.002
1056-4993/13/$ – see front matter © 2013 Elsevier Inc. All rights reserved.

conventional medicine. All valid treatments can and should be used by practitioners, so it is often difficult to define what lies outside of conventional medicine. Although the authors use the term CAM extensively in this article, it should be viewed as a kind of misnomer, because the use of this term suggests a definable distinction.

In psychiatry as well, the unconventional treatments of yesterday have become the established treatments of today (eg, cognitive–behavioral therapy). Yet physical exercise and even light therapy remain somewhat marginalized treatments in psychiatry, and they are infrequently prescribed in child and adolescent psychiatry. Music therapy is a common intervention used in the psychiatric inpatient care of youth, but child and adolescent psychiatrists rarely prescribe it for their outpatients. Treatment of psychiatric disorders with micronutrients (vitamins and minerals) may be viewed as unconventional, but these ubiquitous biologic molecules are basic to the understanding of biochemistry and medicine. All of these treatments may look different from usual psychotherapies and psychiatric medications, but does that mean that they should be considered to lie outside of conventional medicine?

Clinicians will find few CAM treatments that are established, which should be expected, by definition. How long would a treatment still be considered unconventional if the data have already proven its efficacy?

The difficulty of drawing firm clinical conclusions from much of the research in CAM psychiatry is comparable to the provisional findings in other fields in medicine and pediatrics. Among the systematic reviews by the Cochrane Collaboration of CAM treatments throughout pediatrics, about 70% of the reviews (109 of 163) have been deemed inconclusive, not permitting firm positive or negative conclusions regarding treatment recommendations.[1] Child and adolescent psychiatrists will nonetheless find a review of these treatments to be clinically useful, because patients and families are often interested in these treatments, and because patients often present situations in which it is helpful to think beyond established evidence-based treatments for a variety of reasons: ineffectiveness of established treatments, lack of medical insurance and financial resources to support conventional treatment, and patient or parent reluctance to employ standard treatments (eg, refusing pharmaceuticals and wanting natural antidepressants).

Researchers, in contemplating the literature on CAM treatments, will find an abundance of opportunities for deepening the evidence base for many interventions that are already supported by encouraging data. CAM offers a cornucopia of possible treatments that cry out for systematic open-label studies and randomized double-blind placebo-controlled studies, with plenty of low-hanging fruit in treatments that appear valuable but have been weakly documented.

Many youths are already being treated with CAM treatments, even if their psychiatrists are unaware of it. There are not good data on this issue in child and adolescent psychiatry, but parents inform pediatricians about their child's use of CAM in only 12% to 44% of cases in the United States.[2–5] Patients expect disinterest, disapproval, or ignorance from physicians regarding CAM treatments.[6] In contrast, the disclosure of CAM treatments to pediatricians is 79% in Germany,[7] where CAM is more supported by professional societies, the government, and the public. Nondisclosure (apart from the trust issues it raises) can be dangerous (eg, in situations where a child is being prescribed a serotonin reuptake inhibitor while a parent administers St. John's wort without telling the prescriber).[8] Such nondisclosure also raises another question. How well can a psychiatrist evaluate the effectiveness of an antidepressant treatment while another antidepressant is being covertly administered in varying doses?

Physicians are not legally obligated to inform patients or families about therapy options that are deemed outside the range of conventional treatment (see the article by

Cohen and colleagues elsewhere in this issue for further exploration of this topic). However, this fact should be only slightly reassuring. In view of the arbitrariness of the distinction between CAM and conventional medicine, clinicians may differ about what CAM treatments need to be described in the process of obtaining informed consent. Should sugar restriction or neurofeedback be discussed before prescribing a psychostimulant for attention-deficit/hyperactivity disorder (ADHD)? Should omega-3 fatty acids be routinely offered as adjunctive treatment for ADHD? For youths with autism, is it still legitimate to skip discussing micronutrients (vitamins and minerals) and omega-3 fatty acids, and when should one present N-acetyl-cysteine in obtaining informed consent? Should light therapy and exercise be discussed as part of consent discussions before a patient is started on an antidepressant? Some parents want to be informed about such options, and some youths do too.

Many of these CAM treatments can be used adjunctively with standard treatments (ie, complementary and integrative medicine). The use of low-risk low-cost adjunctive treatments may be defensible even when the level of data supporting their use is not compelling. Adding physical exercise to the regimen of an adolescent with depression, or omega-3 fatty acids for a child with ADHD or autism, might be sensible based on positive open trials or just 1 randomized controlled trial (and not just because of their putative benefits for general health).

Readers should be cautioned that adverse effects of CAM treatments tend to be under-reported in many publications in the medical literature (let alone the lay media). In some reports, adverse effects are not systematically assessed or might not even be mentioned.

CAM has been particularly advanced in Germany,[9] and the US government has become quite active in promoting the development of CAM. New research on CAM is greatly aided by the National Institutes of Health through the National Center for Complementary and Alternative Medicine (NCCAM) and the Office of Dietary Supplements (ODS), which offer funding opportunities and support for the development of this field (see the article by Edwards and colleagues elsewhere in this issue for further exploration of this topic).[7]

The development of CAM is limited by the fact that many of these treatments are not patentable and so do not generate large profits to drive research or marketing. Pharmaceutical advertising is a "conventional" way of influencing physicians' treatment recommendations, and the industrial manufacturing establishment itself creates a sense of legitimacy of novel treatments: In contrast, CAM treatments, even an established natural antidepressant such as S-adenosylmethionine, cannot compete at this level. Some physicians may have an internalized suppression of their receptivity to natural products, which they may experience as inferior because they originate outside of conventional medical production by large multinational pharmaceutical houses. This situation is compounded by the low level of government oversight and regulation of the quality and safety of dietary supplements and natural products.

The US Food and Drug Administration (FDA) is often quite forward and progressive, but it is constrained by congressional mandates and legislative funding. Its role in this field has been limited in comparison to its regulation of pharmaceutical agents and medical devices. The FDA does not oversee evaluation of the safety or efficacy of non-pharmaceutical compounds before their marketing, and these products can be marketed without approval by or even registration with the FDA. Manufacturers are solely responsible for the safety of their products, although the FDA can take action if a product appears unsafe in postmarketing reports of its adverse effects, which manufacturers are required to report to the FDA. Manufacturers also have considerable freedom in the labeling and advertising of their products. They may not make claims about treating specific medical diseases, but they can make general health claims ("enhances neuron functioning, promotes mental well-being"); however, the FDA does require such claims to be accompanied by a notice on the bottle saying, "These statements have not been evaluated by the Food and Drug Administration. This product is not intended to diagnose, treat, cure, or prevent any disease." Certain compounds are designated by the FDA to be "generally recognized as safe" (GRAS) based on scientific data. Overall, the role of the FDA in regulating dietary supplements is quite narrow compared with its supervision of rigorous premarket testing of the efficacy and safety of pharmaceuticals, its oversight of pharmaceutical product quality, its tight monitoring of the wording in package inserts, and its strict regulation of advertising in medical journals and public media.

This lower level of governmental oversight means that products sold might, in some instances, contain none of the ingredients that they are labeled as containing. The public is not necessarily aware that there is no safety testing of health food store products nor oversight of quality control. Prescribers who use these natural products and dietary supplements will want to become familiar with specific brands and products. In general, it is probably advisable to stick with major brands that have been generally reliable (which include, in alphabetical order, Gaia, GNC, Jarrow, Pure Encapsulations, Solgar, TwinLab, Vitamin Shoppe, Vitamin World, among many others). ConsumerLab.com is a helpful resource for obtaining specific information about different companies and their products, and for following general developments in this area. Many of these products are available at health food stores, but prescribers can inform patients that certain online sources offer brand name products at discounted prices (eg, Vitacost.com, LuckyVitamin.com, Amazon.com).

Health insurance companies often appear more anti-CAM than physicians. Most physicians at least entertain the possibility that some CAM treatments may work, but third-party payers have not seemed to realize that it might be worth paying for multivitamins. The lack of reimbursement by insurance companies for an inexpensive efficacious antidepressant like SAMe for adults is clinically illogical and economically self-defeating. To address this problem, efficacy studies and especially pharmacoeconomic studies of CAM treatments are needed. Pharmacoeconomic studies about CAM treatments are increasing but are still extremely limited, and comparative effectiveness studies will be particularly helpful.[10]

Some current data suggest that doctors with additional training in CAM may be able to deliver comparable care with lower health care costs than conventional doctors,[11–13] mainly due to lower rates of hospitalization and pharmaceutical use.[13,14] Interpretation of these findings is complicated by differences in the patient populations seeking CAM treatments. CAM-seeking patients tend to be more educated, more wealthy, and more attentive to healthy lifestyles and preventive care. They may also prefer generally less aggressive conventional care. Although some methodological problems complicate these findings, specific CAM treatments whose data suggest equivalent outcomes with lower costs include acupuncture (for migraine), chiropractic manipulation (for neck pain), spa therapy (Parkinson disease), stress management (patients receiving cancer chemotherapy), nutrient supplementation (patients undergoing gastrointestinal surgery), and biofeedback (irritable bowel syndrome),[15] and CAM treatments may also be cost-effective as part of postsurgical care.[13,16] Some managed care organizations have been providing CAM options for over 15 years. Humana, one of the largest managed care organizations in the United States, created a network of CAM providers 10 years ago, offering its patients a 30% discount on fees.[17]

Incorporation of CAM treatments does not require clinicians to make fundamental changes in their practice. Beginning to use new CAM treatments, learning about available CAM internists or specialists in one's locale, and allowing colleagues to know of one's interest in CAM treatments need not be major steps. Other physicians might make larger steps, such as becoming advocates for CAM in their hospitals and professional societies, teaching colleagues and medical students about using CAM techniques, incorporating naturalistic CAM research studies into their clinical practice, conducting a funded research project, joining an integrative practice, or starting a CAM clinic (see the article by Shannon elsewhere in this issue for further exploration of this topic). Physicians will individually make choices about where they wish to begin. Some will choose to incorporate CAM psychopharmacological approaches; others will delve more deeply into a broader range of holistic treatments.

The American Academy of Child and Adolescent Psychiatry (AACAP) has established its Committee on Integrative Medicine in recognition of parents' and physicians' increasing interest in dietary supplements, natural products, mind–body interventions, and other modalities to enhance the psychiatric treatment of children and adolescents. Parents are motivated by the slow speed and limited efficacy of conventional treatment as well as some very realistic concerns about the adverse effects of psychiatric medications.

A basic question that physicians may ask themselves is: "Does the advent of CAM present me with a conflict of world views, or is it an opportunity for the expansion of my range of influence?" The challenge to individual physicians is whether and how to participate in the emergence of complementary and alternative treatments in medicine. It is helpful to remember that a physician's excessive skepticism as well as excessive enthusiasm can stand in the way of patient care. The low stigma and low costs of many forms of CAM, especially in comparison to many conventional psychiatric treatments, make them attractive to patients and should provoke the interest of physicians.

REFERENCES

1. Meyer S, Schroeder N, Willhelm C, et al. Clinical recommendations of Cochrane reviews in 3 different fields of paediatrics (neonatology, neuropaediatrics, and complementary and alternative medicine): a systematic analysis. Pediatr Int 2013. [Epub ahead of print]. http://dx.doi.org/10.1111/ped.12109.
2. Sawni-Sikand A, Schubiner H, Thomas RL. Use of complementary/alternative therapies among children in primary care pediatrics. Ambul Pediatr 2002;2(2): 99–103.
3. Spigelblatt L, Laîné-Ammara G, Pless IB, et al. The use of alternative medicine by children. Pediatrics 1994;94(6 Pt 1):811–4.
4. Yussman SM, Ryan SA, Auinger P, et al. Visits to complementary and alternative medicine providers by children and adolescents in the United States. Ambul Pediatr 2004;4(5):429–35.
5. Sibinga EM, Ottolini MC, Duggan AK, et al. Parent-pediatrician communication about complementary and alternative medicine use for children. Clin Pediatr (Phila) 2004;43(4):367–73.
6. Adler SR, Fosket JR. Disclosing CAM use in the medical encounter. J Fam Pract 1999;48(6):453–8.
7. Gottschling S, Gronwald B, Schmitt S, et al. Use of complementary and alternative medicine in healthy children and children with chronic medical conditions in Germany. Complement Ther Med 2013;21(Suppl 1):S61–9.
8. Walter G, Rey JM. Use of St. John's Wort by adolescents with a psychiatric disorder. J Child Adolesc Psychopharmacol 1999;9(4):307–11.

9. Joos S, Musselmann B, Szecsenyi J. Integration of complementary and alternative medicine into family practices in Germany: results of a national survey. 2011;2011:495813.

10. Witt CM, Chesney M, Gliklich R, et al. Building a strategic framework for comparative effectiveness research in complementary and integrative medicine. Evid Based Complement Alternat Med 2012;2012:531096.

11. Martin BI, Gerkovich MM, Deyo RA, et al. The association of complementary and alternative medicine use and health care expenditures for back and neck problems. Med Care 2012;50(12):1029–36.

12. Studer HP, Busato A. Comparison of Swiss basic health insurance costs of complementary and conventional medicine. Forsch Komplementmed 2011;18(6): 315–20.

13. Kooreman P, Baars EW. Patients whose GP knows complementary medicine tend to have lower costs and live longer. Eur J Health Econ 2012;13(6):769–76.

14. Sarnat RL, Winterstein J, Cambron JA. Clinical utilization and cost outcomes from an integrative medicine independent physician association: an additional 3-year update. J Manipulative Physiol Ther 2007;30(4):263–9.

15. Herman PM, Craig BM, Caspi O. Is complementary and alternative medicine (CAM) cost-effective? A systematic review. BMC Complement Altern Med 2005;5:11.

16. Kennedy DA, Hart J, Seely D. Cost effectiveness of natural health products: a systematic review of randomized clinical trials. Evid Based Complement Alternat Med 2009;6(3):297–304.

17. McHughes M, Timmermann BN. A review of the use of CAM therapy and the sources of accurate and reliable information. J Manag Care Pharm 2005;11(8): 695–703.

Attention-Deficit/Hyperactivity Disorder: Dietary and Nutritional Treatments

L. Eugene Arnold, MEd, MD[a],*, Elizabeth Hurt, PhD[b],
Nicholas Lofthouse, PhD[c]

KEYWORDS

- ADHD • Treatment • Vitamins • Minerals • Diet • Essential fatty acids • Omega-3
- Sugar

KEY POINTS

- Most ingestible complementary/alternative treatments for attention-deficit/hyperactivity disorder (ADHD) have an inconclusive evidence base, but some are safe, easy, cheap, and sensible (SECS) enough to be tried while awaiting better research.
- With more than a dozen placebo-controlled trials of varying quality, omega-3 (ω-3 or n-3) fatty acids seem to have a small to medium benefit.
- Herbs are essentially crude drugs, mostly without good standardization and quality control. Some may be contaminated with heavy metals. Only one (Pycnogenol) has placebo-controlled evidence of modest effectiveness in ADHD.
- RDA/RDI multivitamin/minerals are reasonable for patients with poor diets, especially with appetite loss from stimulant medication. This may not treat ADHD but can provide nutritional support.

BACKGROUND
Need

The interest in complementary and alternative treatments for ADHD is fueled in part by disappointment with established treatments. Although carefully managed Food and Drug Administration (FDA)-approved medication shows a large benefit for ADHD symptoms for up to 2 years in group data,[1,2] it is not satisfactory for a substantial

Disclosures: L.E. Arnold has had research funding from CureMark, Lilly, and Shire; has been on advisory boards for AstraZeneca, Biomarin, Novartis, Noven, Seaside Therapeutics, and Shire; and had travel support from Noven. E. Hurt has had research funding from Bristol-Meyers Squibb. N. Lofthouse has no financial disclosures.
[a] Nisonger Center, Ohio State University, McCampbell 395E, 1581 Dodd Drive, Columbus, OH 43210, USA; [b] Nisonger Center, Ohio State University, 1581 Dodd Drive, Columbus, OH 43210, USA; [c] OSU-Harding Neuropsychiatry Facility, Ohio State University, 1670 Upham Drive, Columbus, OH 43210, USA
* Corresponding author.
E-mail address: L.Arnold@osumc.edu

Child Adolesc Psychiatric Clin N Am 22 (2013) 381–402
http://dx.doi.org/10.1016/j.chc.2013.03.001
1056-4993/13/$ – see front matter © 2013 Elsevier Inc. All rights reserved.

childpsych.theclinics.com

minority,[3] does not normalize functioning, does not have conclusive evidence of benefit beyond 2 years,[4] and is rejected by a substantial minority of the public. Behavioral treatment, although theoretically longer lasting in effect, is insufficient alone, even in a multicomponent intervention package, in one-fourth of children with moderate to severe combined-type ADHD.[1] Even when combined with medication, behavioral treatment leaves one-third of patients symptomatic.[3] Thus, additional treatment options are needed.

This article reviews common dietary elimination and supplement strategies and the evidence or lack thereof for each strategy. For a more comprehensive review, see Arnold and colleagues.[5] Because most of these strategies do not have compelling, conclusive evidence, such as placebo-controlled randomized clinical trials (RCTs) with clear results, clinical application must depend in most cases on other criteria.

SECS Versus RUDE Criterion

A treatment that is safe, easy, cheap and sensible (SECS) does not need as much evidence to justify an individual patient trial as one that is risky, unrealistic, difficult, or expensive (RUDE).[5] Passing the SECS criterion does not necessarily mean a treatment is evidence-based in the usual sense. The criterion is merely an interim guide awaiting further research.

Dietary Intervention is Mainstream Medicine

Two dietary strategies are currently established in mainstream medicine. The first is to eliminate or restrict; examples include copper in Wilson's disease, phenylalanine in phenylketonuria, and iron in hemochromatosis. The second is to add or supplement, examples of which are iodine for myxedema madness, cyanocobalamin (vitamin B_{12}) for psychosis of pernicious anemia, thiamine (vitamin B_1) for Wernicke's encephalopathy, and niacin (vitamin B_3) for dementia of pellagra.

ELIMINATION OR RESTRICTION OF FOODS OR DIETARY COMPONENTS

A dozen placebo-controlled studies have explored elimination of various foods (wheat, corn, and dairy) or additives (colors, preservatives, and artificial flavors) suspected of a deleterious behavioral effect regarding ADHD symptoms. A few of these studies involved random assignment to elimination diet versus control diet. For example, in a 10-week single-blind crossover study, Kaplan and McNicol[6] supplied whole families with their food: a 3-week baseline followed by a 3-week placebo diet before beginning a 4-week experimental diet. This diet eliminated dyes, flavors, monosodium glutamate, chocolate, caffeine, preservatives, and dairy and allowed only a small amount of sugar. Use of this elimination diet correlated with behavioral and sleep improvement in half of the participants. There was negligible placebo diet effect.

Most studies of elimination/restriction diets involved open trials followed by placebo-controlled challenges with dietary components identified as problematic by open challenge. In a typical study,[7] 78 children openly tried the elimination diet, and 59 (three-fourths) of them improved, but only 47 (four-fifths) of these responders later relapsed with open challenge, suggesting 47/78 (60%) as the upper limit of effective response to the diet. Of the 47 responders, 23 received a placebo-controlled challenge, 19 of whom completed: 14 (three-fourths) of those reacted to the active but not placebo challenge. These 14 placebo-confirmed reactors comprised 18% of the original 78 children, thus setting 18% as the lower limit of response.

Similarly, in a study of 76 children selected for hyperactivity,[8] 62 improved on open oligoantigenic or few foods diet, experiencing fewer headaches, stomachaches, and fits. When 28 of these children entered a double-blind crossover, symptoms returned more often after eating the suspected food or additive than after placebo food/additive. Of 48 foods incriminated, colors and preservatives were the most common.

Rowe and Rowe[9] selected 200 participants of 800 hyperactive children and found that 150 improved openly with elimination of artificial food coloring (food dyes) and deteriorated on open addition of food coloring: 34 of these individuals and 20 controls entered a double-blind challenge with 6 doses of tartrazine (FD&C Yellow 5) and placebo. Of these, 22 of the 34 reactors (65%) and 2 of the 20 controls (10%) reacted to the dye challenge with irritability, restlessness, and sleep disturbance.

Some studies of elimination diets have yielded negative results. For example, David[10] found no reaction in 24 hospitalized children with a history of behavioral effects from tartazine or benzoic acid on double-blind challenge with both.

The Southampton Studies

The Southampton studies reoriented thinking about food colorings from an ADHD problem to a public health problem. In these 3 studies of nonclinical samples (2 studies in preschool children and 1 in school children aged 8 to 9 years),[11–13] children were classified as hyperactive or not (based on a rating scale and other measures) and as atopic or not (based on a skin prick test). The challenge in these studies was mixed fruit juice with or without a 20-mg to 62-mg mixture of dyes (sunset yellow, tartrazine, carmoisine, ponceau 4R, quinoline yellow, and/or allura red AC) and 45 mg of sodium benzoate. Blinding of the taste and appearance was rigorous and effective, confirmed by adult taste panels and parent guesses at the end of the first preschool study.

- The first preschool Southampton study[11] showed a significantly greater increase in hyperactivity (actually all ADHD symptoms) on active challenge with dye (20 mg) than on placebo, assessed by parent ratings, with a small to medium effect. There were no associations with atopy (suggesting that reactions to the food color challenge was not immune mediated) or with high hyperactivity scores.
- The second Southampton study[12] replicated the first study in preschoolers using a composite primary outcome measure.
- The third Southampton study[12] was conducted on 8-year-olds to 9-year-olds using larger doses of dye (separate challenges of 25 mg or 62 mg) that were still within current mean daily consumption. The primary outcome was a composite of neuropsychological measures and parent and teacher ratings. The effect of dye challenge was small but significant and applicable to the whole population, not just those with ADHD syndrome.

Gene Polymorphisms

Gene polymorphisms moderated the effect of dye mixes on global hyperactivity score in the Southampton studies. For both ages, hyperactivity was moderated by a histamine gene (HNMT Thr105Ile). For children ages 8 to 9, but not significantly for the younger children, hyperactivity was also significantly moderated by a different histamine gene (HNMT T939C) and a dopamine gene (DAT1). COMT val108met, ADRA C1291G, and DRD4 rs740373 were not significant.[13] For HNMT T939C, the C allele was protective against dye effect. This allele was present in only 40% of the Southampton sample, leaving 60% of the child population vulnerable to dyes, again underscoring that food dyes (and/or sodium benzoate) are a public health rather than ADHD problem.

More comprehensive elimination diets (such as oligoantigenic regimens) risk exposing children to nutritional imbalances. Additionally, such diets may delay or distract from more effective treatment if continued despite lack of benefit. Such a diet may also precipitate or aggravate parent-child conflict over dietary transgressions and for some may complicate preexisting eating or body image issues. Finally, elimination diets are not cheap or easy and can consume parental time, money, and effort for intensive management. A well-managed elimination diet that restricts unhealthy food choices, supplemented with diet-deficient vitamins and minerals, however, may improve nutrition.

In summary, food and additive sensitivity is not a major cause of diagnosable ADHD but may occasionally be a significant factor. Two weeks of a severely restricted diet should not be exceeded without obvious benefit. If it seems beneficial, foods should be added back one at a time to identify the culprits responsible for any symptoms. Although food dyes are not a major cause of ADHD, their minimization in the diet could benefit the majority of the population.

Sugar

Many placebo-controlled studies, both elimination trials and challenges, have been conducted on sugar. Most have yielded negative results, suggesting that sugar does not cause ADHD and may not even aggravate ADHD symptoms. Sugar is often accompanied, however, by dyes and artificial flavors, and excess sugar has other known health implications. Rarely, a child's concentration problems occur mainly before meals, suggesting hypoglycemic episodes, which could be exacerbated by high sugar meals and relieved by between-meal protein snacks. Reasonable sugar restriction passes the SECS criterion as a general health measure (refined sugar is not an essential food), but it is not an effective treatment of ADHD by itself.

NUTRITIONAL SUPPLEMENTS

The opposite strategy from elimination/restriction is dietary supplementation. Dietary components are typically categorized from a nutritional standpoint as macronutrients or micronutrients, based on the quantities that a healthy diet would contain. Macronutrients include protein/amino acids and essential fatty acids. Micronutrients include vitamins and minerals, especially iron, zinc, and magnesium.

"Eat a Good Breakfast"

A classroom study[14] highlights the importance of breakfast for preventing symptoms of inattention. It is well known that the attention of normal children as well as children with ADHD wanes over the course of the morning at school. In a regular classroom, children given a whole-grain cereal and milk breakfast (containing some protein, minerals, and vitamins) deteriorated less (by approximately half) in their attention than those given no breakfast. The same number of calories in a glucose drink resulted, however, in faster deterioration than the no-breakfast condition, reaching the same eventual peak of inattention (**Fig. 1**). As expected, a decently nourishing breakfast promotes attention compared with a sugary breakfast or no breakfast, but it is unclear whether this benefits ADHD children more than normal children.

Amino Acids

Children with ADHD have been shown to have low levels of certain amino acids[15,16] and also show nitrogen wasting,[17] suggesting poor use of protein. Several essential amino acids are substrate for neurotransmitter production (tryptophan, tyrosine, and phenylalanine). Some short-term benefit for ADHD has been seen from tryptophan, tyrosine, and phenylalanine, but this usually dissipates by 2 months.[18–22]

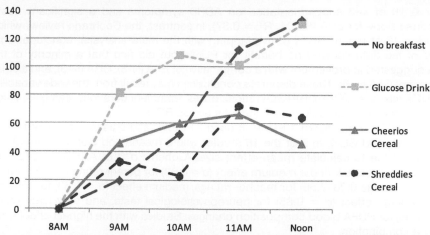

Fig. 1. Deterioration in attention scores (higher score worse) in normal children after different breakfasts at 8:00 AM—Cheerios whole-oat cereal or Shreddies whole-wheat cereal, both consumed with milk. The glucose breakfast had the same number of calories as the cereal breakfasts. Both cereal breakfasts damped the late-morning attention deterioration. (*Data from* Wesnes KA, Pincock C, Richardson D, et al. Breakfast reduces decline in attention and memory over the morning in schoolchildren. Appetite 2003;41(3):329–31.)

There is some risk from toxic catabolic products of increased neurotransmitter turn-over from the supply-side metabolism of increased substrate. S-adenosylmethionine, with a different mechanism (direct dopamine agonist) than the substrate amino acids, showed some promise in a 4-week adult study,[21] but the authors do not know of a longer-term follow-up. A safer approach to maintaining adequate substrate intake and compensating for nitrogen wasting is simply to eat adequate high-quality protein. Processed/refined amino acid supplementation (ie, amino acids not in the natural context of complex proteins) does not currently pass the SECS criterion.

Essential Polyunsaturated Fatty Acids

Omega-3 (ω-3 or n-3) and omega-6 (ω-6 or n-6) polyunsaturated fatty acids (PUFAs) are necessary for neuronal membrane structure, fluidity, and function, providing a nest for receptors, and facilitating electrical transmission. They are also the substrate for production of prostaglandins and other eicosanoids. They are called essential fatty acids because mammalian metabolism cannot synthesize them, so they must be ingested. The main ω-3 acids are eicosapentaenoic (EPA) (20 carbons) and docosahexaenoic (DHA) (22 carbons), which can be derived from α-linolenic (18 carbons) by intact desaturation and elongation metabolism. The main ω-6 acids are γ-linolenic (GLA) (18 carbons) and arachidonic (20 carbons), which can be derived from linoleic (18 carbons) by intact metabolism.

Lower levels of both ω-3 and ω-6 have been observed in ADHD compared with controls.[23–25] Severity of ADHD symptoms in children correlated with lower ω-3 and/or higher ω-6 levels.[26,27] When manipulated in laboratory animals, ω-3 deficiency has led to hyperactivity and decreased visual attention.

To date, there have been 16 published placebo-controlled RCTs in children with ADHD diagnoses or symptoms,[25,28–45] 1 meta-analysis,[46] and 1 Cochrane review.[47] The meta-analysis (10 of the 16 RCTs) found a significant ($P<.0001$) but small effect (g = 0.31) of ω-3 supplementation on ADHD symptoms and a significant dose-response slope for EPA ($P<.04$, $R^2 = 0.37$). In contrast, the Cochrane review, which included 13 of the 16 RCTs (7 overlapping with the meta-analysis), concluded that most of the data showed no benefit for PUFAs but did find that a minority of the data suggested improvement with a combination of EPA (ω-3), DHA (ω-3), and a small amount of GLA (ω-6). These disparate conclusions may result from the wide variability of PUFA mixes (eg, EPA/DHA/GLA ratios), doses, treatment durations, samples, study designs, and/or methodological limitations across RCTs.

Of 16 RCTs, 3 examined 1 PUFA, 8 used 2 PUFAs, and 5 used 3 or more PUFAs (EPA, DHA, and GLA). In 9 of the 16 studies where means and standard deviations were available to calculate mean effect sizes (Cohen's d[48]) of ADHD-specific outcomes, the authors found a medium effect ($d = 0.63$) for parent ratings, a large effect ($d = 1.04$, range 0.28–2.56) for teacher ratings, medium effect ($d = 0.63$) for clinician ratings, large effect ($d = 0.85$) for neuropsychological tests, and very large effect ($d = 1.56$) for PUFA blood composition changes. Studies with the highest effect sizes used a combination.

PUFAs pass the SECS criterion for treating ADHD and are good for general health as well (**Fig. 2**). EPA may be the most important PUFA, but there have been no studies of EPA monotherapy, so it is reasonable to use a mix of EPA and DHA. Fish oil is a cheap source, costing less than $5 a month. It is important to make sure the product label specifies, "mercury-free" or "USP." An acceptable dose is 1 g to 2 g per day from preschool age and up. At least 3 months should be allowed to see results, and a recent study[45] suggests better results at 6 than at 3 months.

Incorporation of PUFAs into phospholipids may enhance the effect. In an RCT comparing ω-3 (250 mg) as fish oil to ω-3 (250 mg) incorporated into phosphatidylserine, and placebo, ω-3/phosphatidylserine was better than both fish oil and placebo (fish oil was better than placebo). The effect size was large ($d = 1.4$) for ω-3 phosphatidylserine versus placebo.[42] Until replication, the cost-benefit ratio of incorporating ω-3 into phosphatidylserine is not clear.

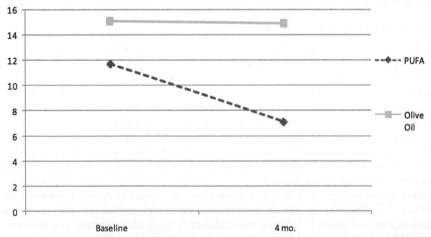

Fig. 2. EPA, DHA, and GLA mix (PUFA) versus olive oil. Teacher-rated inattention on 0–27 scale, $P = .03$. Vertical axis is symptom rating, higher worse. (*Data from* Stevens L, Zhang W, Peck L, et al. EFA supplementation in children with inattention, hyperactivity, and other disruptive behaviors. Lipids 2003;38(10):1007–21.)

Glyconutritional Supplements

Glyconutritional supplements consist of 7 saccharides essential for glycoprotein and glycolipid production and for cell communication. Two open trials reduced parent-rated inattention and hyperactivity/impulsivity ratings significantly by 15% to 25% and sustained the improvement for 6 weeks.[49] This degree of change is probably a placebo response, and a third open trial showed no effect. Glyconutritional supplements do not currently pass the SECS criterion.

Micronutrients: Vitamins/Minerals

Three placebo-controlled multimegavitamin supplementation studies[50–52] found no benefit for ADHD symptoms. Megavitamin doses are several orders of magnitude over the RDA/RDI, such as 1000 mg of a B vitamin or 10 g of vitamin C. Old pilot data[53,54] show promise for specific single megavitamins but have not been pursued. Specific megavitamins could act as drugs instead of vitamins, altering metabolic pathways. Although this area of research warrants carefully controlled exploration, multi-megavitamin dosage poses some risk (eg, hepatoxicity and peripheral neuropathy) and does not currently pass the SECS criterion for clinical use. This needs to be distinguished from more moderate doses, above the RDA/RDI but not generally in the megadosage range, such as the 36-ingredient micronutrient formulation (EMPowerPlus) examined by Rucklidge, who found significant placebo-controlled benefit in adults with ADHD (Julia Rucklidge, PhD, personal communication, 2013).

The RDA/RDI of multivitamin/minerals has not been examined for treating diagnosed ADHD, but there is some collateral evidence from undiagnosed children. Two placebo-controlled studies of unselected schoolchildren[55,56] (total N = 107) showed significant improvement on measures of IQ, attention/concentration, fidgeting, and reaction time in intent-to-treat analysis, although the advantage was restricted to the lower SES in a subgroup analysis. A third study showed no significant effect on reasoning skills. Many children do not eat a balanced diet, even in middle-class families, and this may be aggravated by appetite suppression from FDA-approved stimulants. Therefore, a careful diet history is advisable for all patients, and, if there is any question, RDA/RDI multivitamin/mineral supplementation passes the SECS criterion certainly as a good general health measure but also because of weak but positive evidence from 2 of 3 controlled studies.

Zinc

Zinc is a cofactor for more than 100 enzymes, including many in the brain. It is necessary for melatonin production, and it regulates dopamine production. Both human and animal studies show that hyperactivity and inattention is associated with low levels of zinc. Compared with normal controls, children with ADHD have lower serum levels of zinc ($d = 2.4$, $P<.001$),[57] and serum zinc correlated inversely ($r = -0.45$) with inattention ratings.[58] Two Turkish RCTs of zinc monotherapy[59,60] showed benefit for ADHD, but 1 of them[60] found this effect was observable only in the children of the least educated mothers. An Iranian RCT[61] found adjunctive benefits of zinc when added to standard methylphenidate treatment.

An American pilot RCT[62] randomized 52 children, ages 6 to 14 years, with ADHD (inattentive or combined type) to zinc (15 mg to 30 mg) (as the glycinate) or matched placebo. After 8 weeks of monotherapy, zinc was no more effective than placebo. With the randomization maintained, a standard dose of d-amphetamine was added; in this adjunctive role, zinc was no better than placebo. After the amphetamine dose was optimized for 3 weeks, adjunctive zinc was still no better than placebo. The optimized dose of d-amphetamine, however, was 37% percent lower with zinc (30 mg) than with placebo.

Possible reasons for the difference in results between the American zinc trial and the Middle Eastern trials may include geographic differences in diet (zinc deficiency is endemic in the Middle East), genetic differences, the zinc anion used in the trials (sulfate in Middle East and glycine in American), the zinc dosage (lower used in the American trial), and socioeconomic status of participants (1 Turkish trial found the effect only with low-education mothers, which might speculatively have correlated with nutritional insufficiency).

There may be a food dye interaction with zinc. Ten children with hyperactivity and reported food dye intolerance had lower levels of serum, urine, and nail zinc than 10 normal control children. With tartrazine challenge, serum and saliva zinc declined and urine zinc increased in the hyperactive but not in the control children.[63] This study was replicated in a larger sample examining 47 hyperactive children with parent-reported reactions to dye and 15 age-matched and gender-matched controls. With a 50-mg challenge of tartrazine or sunset yellow, but not with placebo, serum zinc decreased and urine zinc increased in hyperactive but not control children,[64] again suggesting zinc wasting from the dyes. The authors speculate whether FDA-approved medications alter the levels of zinc and other nutrients. The dye-induced changes in zinc levels correlated with behavioral deterioration in both studies. These studies add to the advisability of recommended daily allowance (RDA)/recommended daily intake (RDI) multivitamin/mineral supplementation (including zinc) for children ingesting food dyes, especially those on long-term stimulant treatment.

Zinc in RDA/RDI doses meets the SECS criterion, especially when delivered as part of a balanced vitamin/mineral supplement, but the direct and adjunctive effects of zinc supplementation on ADHD are still unclear.

Magnesium

Polish investigators reported that 34% of a sample of ADHD children were deficient in magnesium as assessed by serum levels (95% if red cell and hair levels were also considered).[65] After 6 months of open supplementation with 200 mg magnesium a day, Conners parent and teacher ratings improved more than for untreated controls, with a large effect size ($d = 1.2–1.4$).[66] The magnesium dosage is important because the dose-response curved is U-shaped; doses exceeding 10 mg/kg/d are toxic. In American samples totaling 166 children, magnesium was normal. It is not clear why American and Polish samples might be different. Magnesium supplementation passes the SECS criterion only in moderate doses (<200 mg/d) or if an individual has serum magnesium levels below the laboratory reference range; in the latter case, magnesium supplementation is standard care, even though the role of magnesium in ADHD remains unclear.

Iron

Iron is the most common mineral deficiency among children. Iron is a necessary coenzyme to synthesize catecholamines, which are considered deficient in ADHD. Iron supplementation of 73 iron-insufficient nonanemic adolescent girls without ADHD improved their verbal learning and memory more than with placebo.[67] Plasma ferritin, a measure of body iron levels, was low in an ADHD sample compared with controls (23 vs 44 ng/mL, $P<.001$) and correlated inversely ($r = -0.3, P = .02$) with Conners parent ratings,[68,69] but the insufficiency may be restricted to comorbid ADHD.[70] In another study of ADHD children, ferritin correlated inversely with optimal amphetamine dose ($r = -0.45$).[71]

There have been only 2 small pilot trials of iron supplementation for ADHD symptoms in drug-free youth. An open trial in 17 nonanemic boys with low iron (ages 7–11) showed improved parent ratings (pre-post $d = 1.0$).[72] In a pilot placebo-controlled randomized study, 23 nonanemic children with ADHD and borderline deficient iron levels were given either ferrous sulfate (80 mg) or placebo for 12 weeks (RDA for iron is 8–15 mg daily). There was a significant decrease in parent-reported ADHD symptoms, with a medium effect size.[69] So 2 pilot studies suggest iron supplementation may help ADHD symptoms in nonanemic youth with low iron.

Iron supplementation beyond the RDA/RDI amount passes the SECS criterion only for patients who have low or deficient iron levels determined by a blood test (because excess iron can risk hemochromatosis). Low ferritin or high transferrin receptor levels confirm iron deficiency or insufficiency, but normal ferritin does not by itself prove normal iron status, because inflammation can artificially raise ferritin. Therefore, C-reactive protein is often ordered with ferritin to check for inflammation. Daily supplementation doses could range from RDA amounts to 50 mg or more per day, depending on the severity of iron insufficiency. Constipation is a side effect, which can be ameliorated by concomitant magnesium. After a few months, the iron level should be rechecked and, if it is normal, the dose should be dropped to an RDA amount. Iron status should be evaluated especially in adolescent girls with ADHD, who are triply vulnerable: growth spurts (preschool or adolescent), dieting fads, and menstruation can deplete iron stores.

METABOLITES
Melatonin

Melatonin is a natural hormone that regulates sleep. Three studies in ADHD youth[73–75] (N = 159), including a placebo-controlled RCT, found significant improvement in sleep onset ($d = .59$–1.02), but no significant improvement in ADHD symptoms. Because the randomized trials were only 10 days to 4 weeks in duration, the possibility that cumulative sleep restoration itself might ameliorate ADHD symptoms in the long run cannot be ruled out. Although not directly effective for ADHD, melatonin passes SECS criteria for treating sleep delay in children with ADHD and might cumulatively alleviate the aggravation of ADHD symptoms resulting from sleep deprivation, but the latter has not been studied.

Dimethylaminoethanol

Dimethylaminoethanol (DMAE), also referred to as deanol or dimethylethanolamine, is believed to be an endogenous precursor of choline and acetylcholine. Low doses of DMAE promote cholinergic neurotransmission, whereas high doses may promote catecholaminergic transmission. A dozen published trials on ADHD include some double-blind RCTs. The best RCT[76] was a 3-arm study comparing DMAE (500 mg), methylphenidate (40 mg), and placebo, which found a significant placebo-controlled effect for both active treatments (DMAE: $d = 0.1$ to 0.6; methylphenidate: $d = 0.8$–1.3). No serious safety problems were reported. The FDA classified DMAE as "possibly effective" for ADHD when it was marketed as a drug. Although significantly less effective than stimulants, DMAE passes the SECS criterion for very mild symptoms or medication refusers, with data supporting a weak effect.

L-Carnitine

L-Carnitine is a metabolite necessary for energy production, ferrying fatty acids into mitochondria. It is also a semiessential nutrient, because most people do not

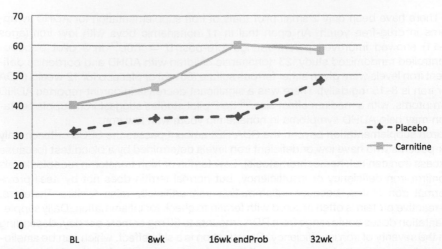

Fig. 3. Timed arithmetic test, with number correct on vertical axis; N = 30, ages 6–12; 15 took L-carnitine, 15 placebo for 16 weeks. At week 16, the placebo group switched to L-carnitine. The carnitine group received L-carnitine throughout. Note delayed effect at 16 weeks, not evident at 8 weeks.

synthesize enough on their own. An Italian RCT of individuals with fragile X syndrome and ADHD showed attentional benefits with L-carnitine supplementation. A Dutch pilot RCT in ADHD of acetyl-L-carnitine (ALC) also showed significant benefit compared with placebo, using an unusual data analysis. Two American RCTs, 1 single site (N = 40) and 1 multisite (N = 112), both failed to show benefit on primary intent-to-treat outcome analysis. There was a significant interaction with ADHD type, however, with inattentive type responding better,[77] and a secondary objective measure of attention (timed arithmetic test) suggested a delayed effect at 4 months (**Fig. 3**). Neither L-carnitine nor ALC is advisable for combined-type ADHD, for which they anecdotally may supply more energy with which to be hyperactive and impulsive, but they pass the SECS criterion for inattentive type with sluggish cognitive tempo, even though the evidence is weak.

Thyroid Hormone

Thyroid hormone is a natural hormone available by prescription to treat hypothyroidism, for which it is standard evidence-based treatment. Generalized resistance to thyroid hormone is a genetic disorder with a high rate of comorbid ADHD syndrome. Inattentive symptoms correlate with high TSH and low T4 levels, and treatment with thyroid supplement improves ADHD symptoms in this rare syndrome. Treatment of any hypothyroid state may help ADHD symptoms.[78,79] Thyroid supplementation passes the SECS criterion only for cases of actual hypothyroidism (signs of which include cold intolerance, coarse hair/skin, sluggish hemodynamics, palpable thyroid, or absent reflexes), which must be confirmed by blood test. When used to treat ADHD symptoms in such cases, thyroid hormone is not a complementary or alternative treatment but standard indicated treatment.

HERBS

Herbal remedies consist of plant parts with pharmacologic activity. They are essentially crude drugs sold over the counter as nutritional adjuncts, and they carry all the risks of drugs, including interactions with other herbs and drugs. Herbal distributors are not required to follow good manufacturing FDA standards, resulting in inconsistent quality and concentrations. Herbal remedies from Asia are often contaminated with toxins, such as lead. They are widely used, but patients often do not inform their doctors of their herb usage.

Pycnogenol

Pycnogenol is an extract of French maritime pine bark. In a small RCT involving 61 children, it improved attention and visual-motor coordination and reduced hyperactivity compared with placebo.[80] Because safety has not been adequately studied, Pycnogenol currently fails the SECS criterion.

Ginkgo Biloba

Ginkgo biloba promotes brain blood flow and inhibits platelet activation. Children (N = 61, ages 6–14) with ADHD were randomized to methylphenidate (20 mg to 30 mg) or Ginkgo biloba (80 mg to 120 mg) for 6 weeks. Methylphenidate yielded significantly better results than Gingko (pre-post d = 1.36 to 1.62 vs 0.52–0.55). By teacher ratings, Ginkgo had no effect. In a safety comparison, methylphenidate resulted in headache, appetite loss, and insomnia more often than Ginkgo,[81] but subdural or anterior eye bleeds have been reported with Ginkgo, so Ginkgo does not pass the SECS criterion.

St. John's Wort

St. John's wort, a serotonergic/noradrenergic/dopaminergic agent, has antidepressant activity. Unmedicated children with ADHD (N = 54, ages 6–17) were given St. John's wort (300 mg) or placebo. No significant difference was observed by parents.[82] Because there are risks (eg, solar sensitivity and serotonin syndrome), St. John's wort does not pass the SECS criterion.

Other Herbs

Other herbs have no evidence supporting use for ADHD symptoms but are still used despite risks. Examples include valerian (headache, mydriasis, restlessness, and cardiac problems), kava-kava (weakness, rash, weight loss, hematuria, increased cholesterol levels, and liver problems), and chamomile (bleeding, vomiting, and hypersensitivity reactions).

HOMEOPATHIC REMEDIES

Homeopathic remedies often include small amounts of herbs. Several studies, including 3 with placebo,[83–85] seemed promising but were flawed in various ways. Furthermore, response took up to 18 months.[85,86] Because of the flaws, equivocal results, and long delay to response, homeopathic remedies fail the SECS criterion because of the risk of delaying proved treatment. Short trials, however, could be defended.

ANTIFUNGAL TREATMENT

An untested hypothesis is that antifungal treatment may improve ADHD symptoms by correcting fungal gut overgrowth causing leaky bowel syndrome. There is some collateral support for this approach from other disorders but no evidence for treating ADHD symptoms. A placebo-controlled trial is needed. This treatment involves some risks and currently fails the SECS criterion.

Table 1
Ingestible complementary and alternative treatments for ADHD reviewed in this article. Level of certainty of research evidence and recommendation grade, before and after slash

Treatment	ADHD Symptoms in Typically Developing Children[a]	Diagnosed ADHD in Children (or Elevated Symptoms Consistent with an ADHD Diagnosis)	Specific Subset of Children with ADHD	Basis for Recommendations for ADHD Symptoms in Youth
Elimination diet	Good/neutral	Good/neutral	Documented reactors: fair/recommend	2 RCTs; 6 placebo-controlled challenges
Sugar restriction	Good/neutral	Good/neutral	—	Meta-analysis
Protein-containing low-sugar breakfast	Fair/recommend	No data	—	1 Controlled trial
Amino acid supplements	—	Fair/recommend against	—	1 RCT with short treatment duration
Polyunsaturated fatty acids (eg, fish oil, ω-3)	—	Good/recommend strongly	—	16 RCTs; meta-analysis
Glyconutritional supplements	—	Poor/insufficient data	—	2 Open trials
Megadoses of vitamins and minerals	—	Fair/recommend against	—	3 RCTs
RDI/RDA multivitamin/mineral supplementation	Fair/Recommend	No data	—	2 Open trials
Zinc supplementation	—	Fair/no recommendation	Children who live in areas with endemic deficiency: fair/recommend	4 RCTs
Magnesium supplementation	—	No data/no recommendation	Children with magnesium deficiency: fair/recommend	3 Open trials
Iron supplementation	—	Poor/Recommend Against	Children with iron deficiency: fair/recommend	1 RCT

Melatonin	—	Fair/recommend against as a treatment of ADHD symptoms	Children with sleep-delay problems: good/recommend	1 RCT; 1 crossover
DMAE	—	Fair/neutral	—	1 PBO-controlled trial with MPH
L-Carnitine or ALC	—	Fair/recommend against for combined-type ADHD	ADHD-I: fair/neutral	2 RCTs
Thyroid supplementation	—	Fair/recommend against	Thyroid abnormality: fair/recommended	1 double-blind crossover
Pycnogenol	—	Fair/neutral	—	1 RCT
Ginkgo biloba	—	Fair/recommend against	—	1 RCT (PBO and MPH)
St John's wort	—	Fair/recommend against	—	1 RCT
Other herbs (eg, valerian, kava-kava, chamomile)	—	No data/recommend against	—	No data
Homeopathic treatments	—	Fair/neutral	—	3 Controlled trials
Antifungal	—	No data	—	No data
Chelation	—	—	Elevated lead levels: fair/recommended	1 RCT

Before each slash: quality of data-based evidence.
After slash: evidence-based clinical recommendation.
United States Preventive Services Task Force (USPSTF) quality of evidence grade (http://www.uspreventiveservicestaskforce.org/uspstf/grades.htm) is a qualitative ranking of the strength of the published evidence in the medical literature regarding a treatment: good, consistent benefit in well-conducted studies in different populations; fair, data show positive effects, but weak, limited, or indirect evidence; and poor, cannot show benefit due to data weakness; no data-no information on youth. USPSTF strength of recommendations: I, insufficient data; D, recommend against (fair evidence of ineffectiveness or harm); C, neutral (fair evidence for but seems risky); B, recommend (fair evidence of benefit and of safety); A, recommend strongly (good evidence of benefit and safety).
Abbreviations: ADHD-I, ADHD, inattentive type; DB, double-blind; MPH, methylphenidate; PBO, placebo.
[a] Note: This column includes only trials in typically developing children that inform understanding of complementary and alternative treatments in youth with ADHD (eg, the Southampton studies on elimination diet). There may be additional trials in typically developing children for purposes unrelated to ADHD.

Table 2
Authors' recommendations and advice/opinion

Treatment	Quality of Evidence for ADHD Symptoms/Clinical Recommendation	Authors' Recommendation, Clinical Tips, and Cautions
Elimination diet	Fair to good/recommended for documented reaction to foods, additives, preservatives. Acceptable for patients without documented reaction.	• Short trial acceptable for patients without documented reaction • Monitor nutritional balance • Monitor family stress of diet implementation (treatment can be difficult to maintain, requires organization and motivation)
Sugar restriction	Good/acceptable, especially if suspicion of prediabetes or diurnal symptom pattern	• Research does not suggest that eliminating sugar decreases ADHD symptoms. • A reduction in sugar can be recommended, however, for all for general health benefit. • Need to monitor parent-child interaction; strict dietary restrictions can lead to parent-child conflict.
Protein-containing, low-sugar breakfast	Fair/recommended	• Recommended for all children, including those with ADHD • Breakfast of whole grains and milk may help maintain attention in AM; however, a high-sugar breakfast may lead to decline in attention.
Amino acid supplements	Poor/recommend against	• Due to lack of research support and metabolic risks, amino acid supplements not recommended. • A diet providing adequate protein is safer and recommended instead.
Polyunsaturated fatty acids (eg, fish oil, ω-3)	Good/recommend strongly	• Definitely recommended for those who do not eat wild oily fish at least 3 times weekly. Sensible for all patients due to general health benefits. • One concern is potential mercury contamination of fish oil. Patients should use mercury-free or USP grade. • May need 3 mo to show effect.
Glyconutritional supplements	Poor/insufficient data	• Given mixed results in open trials, it is not recommended. • Main known risk is the delay of proved treatment.
Megadoses of vitamins and minerals	Fair/recommend against	• Not recommended • Risks include toxicity (eg, liver and peripheral neuropathy) and delay of proved treatment.

(continued on next page)

Table 2 (continued)		
Treatment	**Quality of Evidence for ADHD Symptoms/Clinical Recommendation**	**Authors' Recommendation, Clinical Tips, and Cautions**
RDI/RDA multivitamin/mineral supplementation	Fair/recommend	• Recommended for all children with ADHD but especially for picky eaters or those with stimulant-decreased appetite
Zinc supplementation	Fair/recommend for those with documented deficiency	• Recommended for those with documented deficiency or insufficiency • Monitor >15 mg closely: high doses of zinc may interfere with iron and copper absorption.
Magnesium supplementation	Fair/recommended only for those with documented deficiency or insufficiency (rare in American children)	• Monitor for toxicity if dose >200 mg or >10 mg/kg daily. • May cause diarrhea.
Iron supplementation	Fair/recommend only for those with documented deficiency or insufficiency	• Monitor for toxicity. • Do not supplement above RDA without blood test evidence of deficiency or insufficiency. • May be constipating; consider combining with magnesium.
Melatonin	Good/recommend for treating comorbid sleep problems, not core ADHD symptoms	• Improves sleep, but there is no evidence of improvement for ADHD symptoms. • May be proconvulsant in children with epilepsy
DMAE	Fair/neutral	• DMAE is acceptable for patients with mild symptoms who choose not to take medication or who fail to respond to medication. • Main known risk is the delay of other proved treatments if DMAE is not effective • Benefit of DMAE is less than FDA-approved stimulant medication
L-Carnitine or ALC	Fair/neutral (for patients with ADHD-I)	• Acceptable for patients with ADHD-I • Not advisable for patients with ADHD-combined or ADHD-H/I • Main known risk is the delay of other proved treatments if ineffective. • Requires 4 mo for effect

(continued on next page)

	Table 2 (*continued*)	

Treatment	Quality of Evidence for ADHD Symptoms/Clinical Recommendation	Authors' Recommendation, Clinical Tips, and Cautions
Thyroid supplementation	Fair/recommended as standard medical treatment of those with hypothyroidism; recommend against for those without thyroid abnormality	• Needs monitoring for typical risks associated with treatment of thyroid dysfunction • Check thyroid function by blood test if cold intolerance, absent, or sluggish reflexes or hypodynamics.
Pycnogenol	Fair/neutral	• Acceptable if other treatments have failed • May contain contaminants • Risks are not adequately studied.
Ginkgo biloba	Fair/recommend against	• Risks include subdural or eye-bleeds • May contain contaminants
St John's wort	Fair/recommend against	• Risks include solar sensitivity and serotonin syndrome • May be useful for depression but not ADHD.
Other herbs (eg, valerian, kava-kava, chamomile)	No data/recommend against	• Not recommended • Risks include cardiac and liver toxicity • May contain contaminants
Homeopathic treatments	Fair/neutral	• Short trials can be defended, although may require 18 mo of treatment for benefit. • Thus, main risk is delay of other treatment.
Antifungal	No data	• Not recommended • Risks are unclear; more research necessary
Chelation	Fair/recommended only if child has elevated lead levels	• Only recommended for those with elevated levels of heavy metals, for which it is standard treatment • Standard risks of chelation treatment apply.

Note: Second column rates United States Preventive Services Task Force quality of evidence/strength of recommendation, third column is personal opinion/general recommendation/clinical tips/cautions.

Abbreviation: USP, US Pharmacopeia.

CHELATION FOR SUBCLINICAL LEAD TOXICITY

Lead burden can result in several kinds of cognitive impairment, including symptoms involving attention and impulse control. When 44 hyperactive children with documented lead toxicity (lead concentration above 25 µg/dL) were randomized to penicillamine, placebo, or methylphenidate for 12 weeks, pencillamine was more effective than placebo ($d = 1.6$) on teacher-rated hyperactivity and was nominally better than methylphenidate (5–40 mg).[87,88] A prevention study with infants was a failed trial. Because of the risks of this treatment, it is contraindicated with normal lead levels but passes the SECS criterion for those with elevated lead levels, for whom it could be considered standard medical treatment.

SUMMARY AND CONCLUSION
Clinical Conclusions

Many complementary/alternative treatments for ADHD are not specific treatments of ADHD but instead sensible health measures. Some are just standard recommendations made for personalized comprehensive medical management, such as iron for deficiency, elimination diet for known sensitivity to food or additives, and treatment of thyroid abnormality or lead burden. Some treatments are good for general health, and possibly or probably have direct or indirect value for treating ADHD, such as ω-3 fatty acids, minimizing food dyes and sugar intake, and RDA/RDI multivitamin/mineral supplementation for individuals with poor diets. Some complementary/alternative treatments are potentially risky, such as amino acids in large quantities, multimegavitamins, some herbs, and antifungals. Many simply do not have enough evidence to form a conclusion about effects on ADHD.

It is necessary to conduct a careful diet history, other history, examination, and sometimes laboratory tests. Most complementary/alternative treatments can be used with established treatment. **Tables 1** and **2** may be useful references for clinicians in educating patients and their families regarding available evidence for treatments in which they express an interest. Note that an important risk for any unproved treatment is delay of proved treatment if substituted.

Promising Research Directions

A placebo-controlled RCT of RDA/RDI multivitamins/minerals in diagnosed ADHD would be fairly easy and cheap to conduct and could have great public health implications. Similarly, RCTs of antifungal therapy and various minerals (especially zinc, iron, and magnesium) would be informative. Seasonal tracking of vitamin D, along with an RCT of vitamin D supplementation should be enlightening, with dosage as one of the issues to be addressed. It would be useful to have an RCT of L-carnitine, specifically focused on the inattentive type of ADHD. A nutritional package of essential fatty acids, RDA/RDI vitamins/minerals, adequate protein, probiotics, sugar moderation, dye minimization, and minimization of ω-6 fatty acids should be compared with a placebo package of interventions of equal intensity over a several-month period and compared with medication. Another useful RCT would be a personalized approach, in which various vitamins, minerals, and essential fatty acids are tested (especially vitamin D, iron, zinc, and magnesium) and a customized nutritional plan compared with a placebo plan of equal complexity.

Such treatment approaches are already widely used without adequate evidence regarding efficacy or safety. Because these interventions are not patentable and, therefore, not attractive for generous industry funding, nutritional interventions should be given priority by federal funding agencies and private foundations.

REFERENCES

1. The MTA Cooperative Group. Moderators and mediators of treatment response for children with attention-deficit/hyperactivity disorder. Arch Gen Psychiatry 1999;56:1088–96.

2. The MTA Cooperative Group. The NIMH MTA follow-up: 24-month outcomes of treatment strategies for Attention-Deficit/Hyperactivity Disorder (ADHD). Pediatrics 2004;113(4):754–61.

3. Swanson JM, Kraemer HC, Hinshaw SP, et al. Clinical relevance of the primary findings of the MTA: success rates based on severity of ADHD and ODD symptoms at the end of treatment. J Am Acad Child Adolesc Psychiatry 2001;40:168–79.

4. Jensen PS, Arnold LE, Swanson J, et al. Follow-up of the NIMH MTA study at 36 months after randomization. J Am Acad Child Adolesc Psychiatry 2007;46(8): 988–1001.

5. Arnold LE, Hurt E, Mayes T, et al. Ingestible alternative and complementary treatments for ADHD. In: Hoza B, Evans SW, editors. Treating attention-deficit disorder. Kingston (NJ): Civic Research Institute; 2011. p. 14-1–14-40.

6. Kaplan BJ, McNicol J. Dietary replacement in preschool-aged hyperactive boys. Pediatrics 1989;83(1):7–17.

7. Carter CM, Urbanowicz M, Hemsley R, et al. Effects of a few food diet in attention deficit disorder. Arch Dis Child 1993;69(5):564–8.

8. Egger J, Graham PJ, Carter CM, et al. Controlled trial of oligoantigenic treatment in the hyperkinetic syndrome. Lancet 1985;1:540–5.

9. Rowe KS, Rowe KJ. Synthetic food coloring and behavior: a dose response effect in a double-blind, placebo-controlled, repeated-measures study. J Pediatr 1994;125:691–8.

10. David TJ. Reactions to dietary tartrazine. Arch Dis Child 1987;62(2):119–22.

11. Bateman B, Warner JO, Hutchinson E, et al. The effects of a double blind, placebo controlled, artificial food colourings and benzoate preservative challenge on hyperactivity in a general population sample of preschool children. Arch Dis Child 2004;89:506–11.

12. McCann D, Barrett A, Cooper A. Food additives and hyperactive behaviour in 3-year-old and 8/9-year-old children in the community: a randomized, double-blind, placebo-controlled trial. Lancet 2007;370:1560–7.

13. Stevenson J, Sonuga-Barke E, McCann D, et al. The role of histamine degradation gene polymorphisms in moderating the effects of food additives on children's ADHD symptoms. Am J Psychiatry 2010;167(9):1108–15.

14. Wesnes KA, Pincock C, Richardson D, et al. Breakfast reduces decline in attention and memory over the morning in schoolchildren. Appetite 2003;41(3):329–31.

15. Bernstein AL. Vitamin B6 in clinical neurology. Ann N Y Acad Sci 1990;585: 250–60.

16. Baker GB, Bornstein RA, Rouget AC, et al. Phenylethylaminergic mechanisms in attention-deficit disorder. Biol Psychiatry 1991;29:15–22.

17. Stein TP, Sammaritano AM. Nitrogen metabolism in normal and hyperkinetic boys. Am J Clin Nutr 1984;39:520–4.

18. Nemzer E, Arnold LE, Votolato NA, et al. Amino acid supplementation as therapy for attention deficit disorder (ADD). J Am Acad Child Adolesc Psychiatry 1986; 25(4):509–13.

19. Reimherr FW, Wender PH, Wood DR, et al. An open trial of l-tyrosine in the treatment of attention deficit disorder, residual type. Am J Psychiatry 1987;144: 1071–3.

20. Wood DR, Reimherr FW, Wender PH. Treatment of attention-deficit disorder with dl-phenylalanine. Psychiatry Res 1985;16:21–6.

21. Shekim WO, Antun F, Hanna GL, et al. S-adenosyl-L-methionine (SAM) in adults with ADHD, RS: preliminary results from an open trial. Psychopharmacol Bull 1990;26:249–53.

22. Wood DR, Reimherr FW, Wender PH. Amino acid precursors for the treatment of attention-deficit disorder, residual type. Psychopharmacol Bull 1985;21:146–9.
23. Mitchell EA, Lewis S, Cutler DR. Essential fatty acids and maladjusted behavior in children. Prostaglandins Leukot Med 1983;12:281–7.
24. Mitchell EA, Aman MG, Turbott SH, et al. Clinical characteristics and serum essential fatty acid levels in hyperactive children. Clin Pediatr 1987;26:406–11.
25. Stevens L, Zhang W, Peck L, et al. EFA supplementation in children with inattention, hyperactivity, and other disruptive behaviors. Lipids 2003;38(10):1007–21.
26. Milte C, Sinn N, Howe P. Polyunsaturated fatty acid status in attention deficit hyperactivity disorder, depression, and Alzheimer's disease: towards an omega-3 index for mental health? Nutr Rev 2009;67(10):573–90.
27. Milte C, Sinn N, Street SJ, et al. Erthrocyte polyunsaturated fatty acid status, memory, cognition, and mood in older adults with mild cognitive impairment and healthy controls. Prostaglandins Leukot Essent Fatty Acids 2011;84:153–61.
28. Aman MG, Mitchell EA, Turbott SH. The effects of essential fatty acid supplementation by Efamol in hyperactive children. J Abnorm Child Psychol 1987;15(1):75–90.
29. Arnold LE, Kleykamp D, Votolato NA, et al. Gamma-linolenic acid for attention-deficit hyperactivity disorder: placebo-controlled comparison to D-amphetamine. Biol Psychiatry 1989;25(2):222–8.
30. Arnold LE, Kleykamp D, Votolato N, et al. Potential link between dietary intake of fatty acids and behavior: pilot exploration of serum lipids in attention deficit hyperactivity disorder. J Child Adolesc Psychopharmacol 1994;4(3):171–82.
31. Voigt RG, Llorente AM, Jensen CL, et al. A randomized, double-blind, placebo-controlled trial of docosahexaenoic acid supplementation in children with attention-deficit/hyperactivity disorder. J Pediatr 2001;139(2):189–96.
32. Brue AW, Oakland TD, Evans RA. The use of a dietary supplement combination and an essential fatty acid as an alternative and complementary treatment for children with attention-deficit/hyperactivity disorder. Sci Rev Alternative Med 2001;5(4):187–94.
33. Richardson AJ, Puri BK. A randomized double-blind, placebo controlled study of the effects of supplementation with highly unsaturated fatty acids on ADHD-related symptoms in children with specific learning difficulties. Prog Neuropsychopharmacol Biol Psychiatry 2002;26(2):233–9.
34. Hirayama S, Hamazaki T, Terasawa K. Effect of docosahexaenoic acid-containing food administration on symptoms of attention-deficit/hyperactivity disorder—a placebo-controlled double-blind study. Eur J Clin Nutr 2004;58(3):467–73.
35. Richardson AJ, Montgomery P. The Oxford-Durham Study: a randomized, controlled trial of dietary supplementation with fatty acids in children with developmental coordination disorder. Pediatrics 2005;115(5):1360–6.
36. Sinn N, Bryan J. Effect of supplementation with polyunsaturated fatty acids and micronutrients on learning and behavior problems associated with child ADHD. J Dev Behav Pediatr 2007;28(2):82–91.
37. Sinn N, Bryan J, Wilson C. Cognitive effects of polyunsaturated fatty acids in children with attention deficit hyperactivity disorder symptoms: a randomised controlled trial. Prostaglandins Leukot Essent Fatty Acids 2008;78(4–5):311–26.
38. Belanger SA, Vanasse M, Spahis S, et al. Omega-3 fatty acid treatment of children with attention-deficit hyperactivity disorder: a randomized, double-blind, placebo-controlled study. Paediatr Child Health 2009;14(2):89–98.

39. Johnson M, Ostlund S, Fransson G, et al. Omega-3/omega-6 fatty acids for attention deficit hyperactivity disorder: a randomized placebo-controlled trial in children and adolescents. J Atten Disord 2009;12(5):394–401.

40. Johnson M, Månsson JE, Ostlund S, et al. Fatty acids in ADHD: plasma profiles in a placebo-controlled study of Omega 3/6 fatty acids in children and adolescents. Atten Defic Hyperact Disord 2012;4(4):199–204.

41. Raz R, Carasso RL, Yehuda S. The influence of shortchain essential fatty acids on children with attention-deficit/hyperactivity disorder: a double-blind placebo-controlled study. J Child Adolesc Psychopharmacol 2009;19(2):167–77.

42. Vaisman N, Kaysar N, Zaruk-Adasha Y, et al. Correlation between changes in blood fatty acid composition and visual sustained attention performance in children with inattention: effect of dietary n-3 fatty acids containing phospholipids. Am J Clin Nutr 2008;87(5):1170–80.

43. Gustafsson PA, Birberg-Thornberg U, Duchén K, et al. EPA supplementation improves teacher-rated behaviour and oppositional symptoms in children with ADHD. Acta Paediatr 2010;99(10):1540–9.

44. Manor I, Magen A, Keidar D, et al. The effect of phosphatidylserine containing omega3 fatty-acids on attention-deficit hyperactivity disorder symptoms in children: a double-blind placebo-controlled trial, followed by an open-label extension. Eur Psychiatry 2012;27:335–42.

45. Perera H, Jeewandara KC, Seneviratne S, et al. Combined w3 and w6 Supplementation in Children With Attention-Deficit Hyperactivity Disorder ADHD) Refractory to Methylphenidate Treatment: a Double-Blind, Placebo-Controlled Study. J Child Neurol 2012;27:747.

46. Bloch MH, Qawasmi A. Omega-3 fatty acid supplementation for the treatment of children with attention-deficit/hyperactivity disorder symptomatology: systematic review and meta-analysis. J Am Acad Child Adolesc Psychiatry 2011;50(10):991–1000.

47. Gillies D, Sinn JK, Lad SS, et al. Polyunsaturated fatty acids (PUFA) for attention deficit hyperactivity disorder (ADHD) in children and adolescents. Cochrane Database Syst Rev 2012;(7):CD007986.

48. Cohen J. Statistical power analysis for the behavioral sciences. 2nd edition. Hillsdale (NJ): Lawrence Earlbaum Associates; 1988.

49. Dykman KD, McKinley R. Effect of glyconutritionals on the severity of ADHD. Proceedings Fisher Institute for Medical Research 1997;1(1):24–5.

50. Arnold LE, Christopher J, Huestis RD, et al. Megavitamins for minimal brain dysfunction: a placebo-controlled study. JAMA 1978;240(24):2642–3.

51. Haslam RH, Dalby JT, Rademaker AW. Effects of megavitamin therapy on children with attention deficit disorders. Pediatrics 1984;74:103–11.

52. Kershner J, Hawke W. Megavitamins and learning disorders: a controlled double-blind experiment. J Nutr 1979;159:819–26.

53. Coleman M, Steinberg G, Tippett J, et al. A preliminary study of the effect of pyridoxine administration in a subgroup of hyperkinetic children: a double-blind crossover comparison with methylphenidate. Biol Psychiatry 1979;14:741–51.

54. Brenner A. The effects of megadoses of selected B complex vitamins on children with hyperkinesis; controlled studies with long-term follow-up. J Learn Disabil 1982;15:258–64.

55. Benton D, Roberts G. Effect of vitamin and mineral supplementation on intelligence of a sample of schoolchildren. Lancet 1988;1(8578):140–3.

56. Benton D, Cook R. Vitamin and mineral supplements improve the intelligence scores and concentration of six-year-old children. Pers Individ Dif 1991;12: 1151–8.
57. Bekaroglu M, Yakup A, Yusof G. Relationships between serum free fatty acids and zinc and ADHD. J Child Psychol Psychiatry 1996;37:225–7.
58. Arnold LE, Bozzolo H, Hollway J. Serum zinc correlates with parent/teacher-rated inattention in children with attention-deficit/hyperactivity disorder. J Child Adolesc Psychopharmacol 2005;15(4):628–36.
59. Bilici M, Yildirim F, Kandil S, et al. Double -blind, placebo controlled study of zinc sulfate in the treatment of attention deficit hyperactivity disorder. Prog Neuropsychopharmacol Biol Psychiatry 2004;28(1):181–90.
60. Uckardes Y, Ozmert EN, Unal F, et al. Effects of zinc supplementation on parent and teacher behaviour rating scores in low socioeconomic level Turkish primary school children. Acta Paediatr 2009;98:731–6.
61. Akhondzadeh S, Mohammadi M, Khademi M. Zinc sulfate as an adjunct to methylphenidate for the treatment of attention deficit hyperactivity disorder in children: a double blind and randomized trial. BMC Psychiatry 2004;4:9.
62. Arnold LE, DiSilvestro RA, Boz zolo D. Zinc for attention-deficit/hyperactivity disorder: placebo-controlled double-blind pilot trial alone and combined with amphetamine. J Child Adolesc Psychopharmacol 2011;21(1):1–19.
63. Ward NI, Soulsbury KA, Zettel VH, et al. The influence of the chemical additive tartrazine on the zinc status of hyperactive children: a double-blind placebo-controlled study. J Nutr Environ Med 1990;1(1):51–8.
64. Ward NI. Assessment of chemical factors in relation to child hyperactivity. J Nutr Environ Med 1997;7(4):333–42.
65. Kozielec T, Starobrat-Hermelin B. Assessment of magnesium levels in children with ADHD. Magnes Res 1997;10:143–8.
66. Starobrat-Hermelin B, Kozielec T. The effects of magnesium physiological supplementation on hyperactivity in children with ADHD: positive response to magnesium oral loading test. Magnes Res 1997;10:149–56.
67. Bruner AB, Joffe A, Duggan AK, et al. Randomized study of cognitive effects of iron supplementation in non-anemic iron-deficient girls. Lancet 1996;348(9033): 992–6.
68. Cortese S, Konofal E, Bernadina BD, et al. Sleep disturbances and serum ferritin levels in children with attention deficit/hyperactivity disorder. Eur Child Adolesc Psychiatry 2009;18(7):393–9.
69. Konofal E, Cortese S, Marchand M, et al. Impact of restless legs syndrome and iron deficiency on attention-deficit/hyperactivity disorder in children. Sleep Med 2007;8(7–8):711–5.
70. Oner D. Supporting students' participation in authentic proof activities in computer supported collaborative learning (CSCL) environments. International Journal Computer Supported Collaborative Learning 2008;3(3):343–59.
71. Calarge C, Farmer C, DiSilvestro R, et al. Serum ferritin and amphetamine response in youth with attention-deficit/hyperactivity disorder. J Child Adolesc Psychopharmacol 2010;20(6):495–502.
72. Sever Y, Ashkenazi A, Tyano S, et al. Iron treatment in children with attention deficit hyperactivity disorder: a preliminary report. Neuropsychobiology 1997; 35:178–80.
73. Tjon Pian Gi CV, Broeren JP, Starreveld JS, et al. Melatonin for sleeping disorders in children with attention deficit/hyperactivity disorder: a preliminary open label study. Eur J Pediatr 2003;162:554–5.

74. van der Heiiden KB. Effect of melatonin on sleep, behavior, and cognition in ADHD and chronic sleep-onset insomnia. J Am Acad Child Adolesc Psychiatry 2007;46(2):233–41.

75. Weiss MD, Wasdell MB, Bomben MM, et al. Sleep hygiene and melatonin treatment for children and adolescents with ADHD and initial insomnia. J Am Acad Child Adolesc Psychiatry 2006;45(5):513–9.

76. Lewis JA, Young R. Deanol and Methylphenidate in minimal brain dysfunction. Clin Pharmacol Ther 1975;17(5):534–40.

77. Arnold LE, Amato A, Bozzolo H, et al. Acetyl-L-carnitine (ALC) in attention-deficit/hyperactivity disorder: a multi-site, placebo-controlled pilot trial. J Child Adolesc Psychopharmacol 2007;17(6):791–802.

78. Álvarez-Pedrerol M, Ribas-Fitol N, Torrent M, et al. TSH concentration within the normal range is associated with cognitive function and ADHD symptoms in healthy preschoolers. Clin Endocrinol 2007;66:890–8.

79. Stein MA, Weiss RE. Thyroid function tests and neurocognitive functioning in children referred for attention deficit/hyperactivity disorder. Psychoneuroendocrinology 2003;28:304–16.

80. Trebaticka J, Kopasova S, Hradecna Z, et al. Treatment of ADHD with French maritime pine bark extract, Pycnogenol. Eur Child Adolesc Psychiatry 2006; 15:329–35.

81. Salehi B. Ginkgo biloba for Attention-Deficit/Hyperactivity Disorder in children and adolescents: a double blind, randomized controlled trial. Prog Neuropsychopharmacol Biol Psychiatry 2010;34:76–80.

82. Weber W, Steop AV, McCarty RL, et al. Hypericum perforatum (St John's Wort) for attention-deficit/hyperactivity disorder in children and adolescents: a randomized controlled trial. JAMA 2008;299(22):2633–41.

83. Strauss LC. The efficacy of a homeopathic preparation in the management of attention deficit hyperactivity disorder. Journal Biomedical Therapy 2002; 18(2):197–201.

84. Lamont J. Homeopathic treatment of attention deficit hyperactivity disorder. Br Homeopath J 1997;86:196–200.

85. Frei H, Everts R, Ammon K, et al. Homeopathic treatment of children with attention-deficit hyperactivity disorder: a randomised, double blind, placebo controlled crossover trial. Eur J Pediatr 2005;164:758–67.

86. Jacobs J, Williams AL, Girard C, et al. Homeopathy for attention-deficit/hyperactivity disorder: a pilot randomized-controlled trial. J Altern Complement Med 2005;11(5):799–806.

87. David OJ, Hoffman SP, Clark J, et al. The relationship of hyperactivity to moderately elevated lead levels. Arch Environ Health 1983;38:341–6.

88. Dietrich KN, Ware JH, Salganik M, et al. Effect of chelation therapy on the neuropsychological and behavioral development of lead-exposed children after school entry. Pediatrics 2004;114(1):19–26.

Mood Disorders in Youth
Exercise, Light Therapy, and Pharmacologic Complementary and Integrative Approaches

Charles W. Popper, MD*

KEYWORDS

- Complementary and alternative medicine • Mood disorders
- Children and Adolescents • Physical exercise • Light therapy • St. John's wort
- S-adenosylmethionine • 5-hydroxytryptophan

KEY POINTS

- Several complementary and alternative medicine (CAM) antidepressant treatments seem promising, based on early data and a few controlled trials.
- Physical exercise may have a mild to moderate effect on mood in adolescents with major depressive disorder (MDD) and in nonclinical youths (effect size 0.3–0.6); aerobics seem only slightly better than muscle-building or stretching.
- Light therapy might help mild or moderate MDD and delayed sleep-phase disorder (a condition that mimics depression).
- Hypericum (St. John's wort) looks tentatively promising; adverse effects and drug interactions are comparable to pharmaceutical antidepressants, but have higher product variability and unpredictability.
- S-adenosylmethionine, established as efficacious in adults, and 5-hydroxytryptophan, a hyperselective serotonergic agent, have received little or no study in youth, despite encouraging anecdotes.
- CAM antidepressants are attractive to the public because they are inexpensive, usually have few adverse effects (except hypericum), and carry little stigma.

INTRODUCTION

Most adults with severe depression use complementary and alternative medicine (CAM) to manage their depressive symptoms.[1,2] Among the 54% of adults with depression who use CAM, 67% also see a psychiatrist for treatment of their

Disclosures: Dr C. Popper is an unpaid consultant to Truehope Nutritional Support and to NutraTek Health Innovations.
None of the agents discussed in this article have marketing approval for psychiatric uses by the US Food and Drug Administration.
Child and Adolescent Psychiatry, McLean Hospital and Harvard Medical School, Belmont, MA 02478, USA
* 385 Concord Avenue, Suite 204, Belmont, MA 02478-3037, USA.
E-mail address: ChasPopper@harvard.edu

depression.[1] Yet only 20% of patients tell their psychiatrists about their CAM treatment.[2,3] No comparable data are available for children with mood disorders, but usage patterns in CAM pediatrics typically follow parents' personal usage.[4–8]

Child and adolescent psychiatrists need to be aware that they cannot assess the effects of conventional medication treatments in their patients unless they are familiar with and monitor changes in concurrent CAM treatments.

For treating major depressive disorder (MDD) in adults, the Task Force on Complementary and Alternative Medicine of the American Psychiatric Association conducted an exhaustive review in 2010 of the published literature on CAM in psychiatry.[9] Based on the quality of the scientific literature, the Task Force found mostly "promising" results for omega-3 fatty acids, St. John's wort (hypericum), folate, S-adenosylmethionine (SAMe), bright light therapy, physical exercise, and mindfulness psychotherapies for treating depression in adults.

The evidence base supporting CAM psychiatric treatments for children and adolescents tends to be weaker and less convincing than similar data in adults. Nonetheless, there are some promising and intriguing findings in the current data on youth. This article, along with others in a forthcoming issue of *Child and Adolescent Psychiatric Clinics of North America*, reviews the available evidence on a broad range of CAM treatments in order to provide an overview of the current options for treating depression in youth (**Box 1**). Exercise and light therapies are discussed first, which are well known but infrequently used by child and adolescent psychiatrists. Then some CAM psychopharmacologic treatments for youth are reviewed, which may be newer territory for many clinicians.

When the term randomized controlled trial (RCT) is used here, it does not imply that the trial was conducted with blinds, because blinding is difficult for some CAM treatments, such as exercise or light therapy, and it does not imply that the control was a placebo, because controls might be a different type of treatment (flexibility training, relaxation), a lower dose, or a waiting list. RCT means that the trial was randomized and controlled.

Some clinicians might not be familiar with the effect size as a means of describing the strength of an effect, such as the magnitude of the therapeutic benefit of a

---

Box 1
Proposed CAM treatments for depression in youth

- Physical exercise
- Bright light (box) therapy
- Dawn simulation devices
- St. John's wort (hypericum)
- 5-Hydroxytryptophan
- S-Adenosylmethionine
- Folate
- Vitamin D
- Other single micronutrients
- Broad-spectrum micronutrients
- Omega-3 fatty acids (specifically, eicosapentaenoic acid or fish oil)

- EEG biofeedback (ie, alpha asymmetry neurofeedback)
- Mindfulness-based stress reduction
- Transcendental meditation
- Progressive muscle relaxation
- Relaxation therapy
- Massage
- Yoga
- Music therapy
- Acupuncture
- Pet therapy
- Aromatherapy

treatment. Effect size has several technical advantages over other statistical descriptors, such as relative independence from sample size. There are various ways of calculating effect sizes, such as Cohen's d or the standardized mean difference (SMD). As an approximate explanation, an effect size of 0.2 to 0.4 might be considered a small effect, 0.5 to 0.7 is a medium effect, and 0.8 and higher is a large effect (an effect size can exceed 1.0).

The five treatments discussed here are presented in order based on the number of currently available RCTs, from most to least, regarding their antidepressant effects, but not necessarily in the order of their clinical value or promise in youth.

PHYSICAL EXERCISE

The Task Force on Complementary and Alternative Medicine of the American Psychiatric Association found generally positive evidence of physical exercise as an adjunctive therapy to conventional antidepressants in adults with MDD, and some preliminary evidence that exercise monotherapy might be comparable in efficacy to antidepressants and possibly more effective in inducing remission and preventing relapse.[9] Of course, youths with MDD might be more (or less) responsive to physical exercise than adults. A Cochrane review[10] examined 28 RCTs that compared physical exercise with a control condition and found that exercise was moderately helpful for adults with depression (effect size, expressed as SMD, of 0.67); however, when the 4 highest-quality trials were analyzed, only a small benefit of exercise on MDD in adults was identified (effect size SMD 0.31).

Clinical trials on exercise and their treatment implications are considered after a review of the correlative and longitudinal findings on the relationship between mood and exercise in youth. These studies provide some insight into the strengths, limitations, and mechanisms of exercise as a psychiatric treatment.

Cross-Sectional Studies in Nonclinical Samples of Youth

In the general population, numerous cross-sectional studies of youth in community samples have examined the cross-sectional relationship between physical exercise and depressive symptoms, using a wide variety of methodologies and depression rating scales, and often using validated and established measures used in psychiatric research. A review of 108 studies of physical activity in youth in 2000[11] found that increased levels of physical activity were correlated with less depressed mood in adolescents (ages 13–18 years), but this correlation was not found in children (ages 3–12 years).

Since that review, such similar studies have primarily examined adolescents rather than children. Of the 8 more recent cross-sectional studies,[12–19] 5 studies again found significant correlations between physical exercise of varying intensities and fewer depressive symptoms in adolescents. Among the 3 studies in adolescents that did not find a cross-sectional correlation between physical exercise levels and mood[15,16] or moods disorders,[14] 1 reported a significant correlation in young adults (ages 20–24 years; odds ratio [OR] 4.0), although not among adolescents,[14] 1 reported a modest correlation between depressive scores and sedentary behavior (although not physical exercise),[15] and 1 appeared too small to show a statistically significant correlation of this small magnitude.[16] All 3 of the largest studies supported a correlation between physical exercise and reduced depression scores.[12,17,19] A cross-sectional study of 1870 adolescents (ages 14–18 years) found that a lower risk of suicide planning was correlated with more aerobic activity (OR 0.73) and more strengthening/toning exercises (OR 0.64),[12] suggesting that the specific type of physical exercise might not be a critical factor.

The relationship between amount of exercise and depressed mood in adolescents was not simple, as shown in 2 studies: A survey of 5453 community youths (11–17 years old), using the Symptoms Checklist 90, found that low-intensity and moderate-intensity exercise reduced the odds of current depression (OR 0.61) and psychosis (OR 0.54) but also found that high-intensity exercise was a risk factor for binge drinking (OR 1.8), hostility (OR 1.4), and suicidality (OR 1.3).[19] In a study of 380 adolescents (mean age 15 years) with eating disorders, 51% of the patients reported engaging in intense compulsive exercise (mean 22 episodes over 3 months for each patient). This "driven exercise" was associated with eating disorder severity (Spearman ρ = 0.46, P<.001) and with depressive symptoms (as measured by Beck Depression Inventory [BDI], Spearman ρ = 0.33, P<.001), especially in patients with vomiting symptoms.[20] These 2 studies suggest that excessive exercise in adolescents can signify depression or related psychopathology,[21] which might dilute or confound the findings of other studies examining correlations between physical exercise and mood (and mental health in general).

As a group, the correlational studies in adolescents suggest that increased physical exercise is correlated with less depressed mood, possibly in a dose-dependent manner, but that excessive exercise could signify psychopathology. Aerobic exercise seemed to have the strongest correlations with less depressed mood, but other types of exercise were significantly correlated as well. In correlational studies, reduced participation might be a result of depressed mood,[22] rather than the other way around, so that causal inferences about therapeutic benefits of exercise cannot be made.

Longitudinal Studies in Nonclinical Community Samples

Attempts to correlate childhood physical activity levels (or changes over time in activity levels) with later mood states have yielded mixed results. A survey of 2152 community adults (ages 20–97 years) found that self-reported memories of low levels of physical activity during childhood (age <15 years) were associated with increased rates of self-reported depressive illness in adulthood (OR 1.35, P<.04).[23] Although this finding is entirely based on recollection (no rating scales), and although adults with depression might recollect their childhoods in more negative terms, the investigators raise the possibility that low levels of physical activity in childhood might be a risk factor for depression in adulthood. This type of study shows why prospective longitudinal studies are needed.

Several prospective longitudinal studies have been conducted in community samples, again mostly on adolescents, and they show a mixed picture of how physical activity levels and moods correlate and change over time. Three large studies[17,18,24] found that adolescents followed over time (for 1–6 years) showed correlations between earlier low physical activity level (both lower levels of vigorous physical activity and, independently, more sedentary behavior) and higher depression scores later. Two of these studies[17,24] found that changes over time (up or down) in physical exercise level correlated inversely with changes in mood scores. However, 3 other large longitudinal studies did not find such longitudinal effects.[13,15,25] A 10-year prospective study of 1293 adolescents (ages 12–13 years) found that depressive symptoms in young adulthood correlated with contemporaneous moderate to vigorous physical activity, but did not correlate with past physical activity levels.[13] In a similar vein, a prospective study of 860 students with depressive symptoms during high school found that they, 3 years after graduation, were less likely to participate in moderate-intensity physical activity and were less likely to be involved in team sports.[26] Together, these studies suggest that past physical activity has a modest and inconsistent effect on subsequent mood, and that current physical exercise is probably more relevant to current mood.

Longitudinal Data on Youth with MDD

In addition to these studies on depressed mood in the general population, there is a single prospective longitudinal study that examined physical activity effects on well-diagnosed MDD in youth.[24] This 6-year prospective naturalistic study of 496 community adolescents (ages 11–15 years) found that increasing physical exercise was linked to a lower risk for subsequent major or minor depression (assessed by K-SADS [Kiddie Schedule for Affective Disorders and Schizophrenia]); for each additional type of physical activity that an adolescent was engaged with, the relative risk of later major depression decreased by 16%.

In summary, the correlational and longitudinal studies suggest that physical exercise in adolescents in community samples might have modest but significant protective effects against depressive moods and possibly depressive disorders, possibly in a dose-dependent manner, but that current mood is mainly correlated with current activity levels. Interpretation of these findings is confounded by the fact that many individuals, when they become depressed, become less physically active,[22,26] are less likely to engage in effortful activities such as exercise, and are less likely to enjoy their activities. The data are consistent with a bidirectional relationship between physical exercise and mood.[24]

These studies also suggest that physical exercise might have broader mental health benefits as well – not only for mood but also for psychosis, anxiety, binge drinking, eating disorders, and hostility.[19] Again, most of the available longitudinal studies have focused on aerobic exercise, but other types of physical exercise such as stretching or strengthening may be beneficial as well, although perhaps not equally.[12] Conspicuously lacking in these correlational and longitudinal data are studies of pre-adolescent youth.

Exercise as Intervention to Improve Depressed Mood in the General Population

A 2006 Cochrane analysis[27] found that exercise, especially aerobic exercise, may have a small therapeutic benefit in improving depressive symptoms in the community populations of youth. Five randomized studies showed a moderate effect of physical exercise on mood in nonclinical populations of youth (effect size SMD 0.66, $P = .03$) compared with no-intervention control groups, but these studies were viewed as methodologically compromised, and the study populations were too heterogeneous to compare easily.[28–32] Even so, this effect size of 0.66 in the general population of youth compares with an effect size of 0.67 found in a similar Cochrane evaluation[10] of the effects of physical exercise on mood in adults with MDD.

In 5 trials comparing high-intensity and low-intensity exercise in youth, the Cochrane analysis found no effect of exercise intensity on depressive symptoms. This contraintuitive finding raises questions about the adequacy of the evidence database, and the Cochrane review[27] concluded that, given the methodological issues, the effect of exercise as an intervention for reducing depressive moods in community youths is undetermined.

Since the 2006 Cochrane review on youth, 5 more RCTs of physical exercise have been conducted in a variety of community youth samples. A community group of 59 adolescents (ages 18–20 years) with persistent mild to moderate depressive symptoms on the Center for Epidemiologic Studies-Depression (CES-D) scale (CES-D >16) were randomized to exercise (group jogging, mild intensity, 50 minutes, 5 times weekly) or their usual (no jogging) activity for 8 weeks.[33] Half of the sample started with the exercise, and half with no jogging, then crossed over at 8 weeks to the other treatment for another 8 weeks. Participants were not evaluated for major depression, but mean CES-D scores reduced from 21 to 15 (standard deviations not specified, $P<.01$) among the completers. The fact that 10 of 59 (17%) youths did not complete the protocol highlights the difficulty of getting adolescents to sustain a program of physical exercise, even those without serious depressive disorders. Yet, for those youths who were able to maintain the protocol, significant mood improvement was observed from low-intensity to moderate-intensity exercise within 8 weeks.

Another RCT examined 80 community adolescents who were randomized to high-intensity aerobic training (n = 22), moderate-intensity aerobic training (n = 19), flexibility training (n = 19), or a control without protocol exercises (n = 20).[34] Exercisers met for group training in 25-minute to 30-minute sessions twice weekly for 10 weeks, and about 25% of participants dropped out. The completers showed no change in mood scores, but mood was inadequately assessed (only by self-reported Multiple Affect Adjective Check List–Depression), so this study provides useful data regarding physiologic improvement but not regarding mood.

An additional 3 RCTs have assessed the mood effects of exercise in community youth who were overweight (body mass index $\geq$85%ile) and obese ($\geq$95%ile). Among obese adolescents, increased depression scores are correlated with reduced cardiopulmonary fitness ($P<.05$), which itself is correlated with anhedonia in this population.[35]

A study of 207 overweight children (ages 7–11 years) compared 20 and 40 minutes of aerobic exercise daily with a control group.[36] Using the Reynolds Child Depression Scale, the more intense exercise regimen was found to reduce depressive symptoms ($P = .045$) relative to controls. This effect appeared to be partly mediated by an increased sense of self-worth resulting from the exercise. However, the effect on self-esteem was observed in white but not black youths, a finding that was attributed to data suggesting that obesity has less effect on self-esteem in black youth than in white youth.[36,37]

Another RCT examined 81 obese youths (ages 11–16 years), of whom 30% had increased baseline scores on the Children's Depression Inventory (CDI $\geq$13).[38] Moderate aerobic exercise (30 minutes, 3 times weekly for 14 weeks) had no effect of exercise on CDI scores compared with placebo, although there were modest improvements in self-esteem.

A third RCT from Iran[39] examined 152 obese public school adolescents (ages 14–19 years) who were randomized either to a program advocating healthy lifestyle (nutrition, health education, and aerobic exercise for about 40 minutes on 3 days weekly) or to an undefined control group. After 6 weeks, depression scores (on a translated BDI) decreased in both treatment and control groups, and equally in both groups, so this is a negative study regarding mood outcome. Self-esteem was not assessed. The program was judged helpful in reducing body mass index and weight ($P\leq.001$) and increasing knowledge of nutrition ($P<.046$).

Of the 3 RTCs on obese youth in the community, the study on overweight preadolescents[36] showed a significant beneficial effect of exercise on mood, but the 2 studies on obese adolescents[38,39] did not.

The findings on overweight and obese youth cannot necessarily be generalized to the total youth population, but if those 3 studies are combined with the other 2 recent RCTs in the general population, then only 2 of the recent 5 studies in the general youth population showed exercise benefits for mood. Of the 3 negative studies, 1 had clearly inadequate methodology,[34] and 2 were conducted on obese adolescents.

Combined with the 5 earlier RCTs reviewed by Cochrane[27] showing an effect size of 0.66, it is possible to view the current evidence base as suggesting that exercise is moderately helpful for reducing depressed mood in the general youth population, except perhaps for obese adolescents (who might need special measures or lengthier periods to respond than the two 6-week and 14-week studies allowed).

Exercise for Treating Major Depression in Youth

Three early small unblinded RCTs have examined exercise in youths with mixed psychiatric diagnoses, including mood disorders. One study was published[40] and 2 are dissertations that were never published in the peer-reviewed literature.[41,42] The published study of 27 adolescents (mean age 16 years)[40] compared aerobic exercise with a no-intervention control group. Only 11 youths completed the study, and no significant changes were noted in BDI scores. One dissertation on 53 youths (mean age 13 years)[41] compared aerobic exercise (60-minute sessions, 3 times weekly for 8 weeks) at higher and lower intensity with a recreational therapy control group, and found no significant changes in CDI depression scores. Another dissertation[42] examined 19 adolescents (ages 12–18 years) in a similar protocol comparing high-intensity intensity and low-intensity aerobic exercise (but no control group), once again finding no significant difference in BDI depression scores. Although these 3 studies had consistently negative findings, the methodological weaknesses (small size, no blinds, diagnostic heterogeneity) do not allow conclusions regarding exercise effects in youth with depression.

In an uncontrolled study of the feasibility of using physical exercise as a treatment of depression in adolescents, Dopp and colleagues[43] recruited 13 adolescents (5 obese, 5 overweight, 3 normal weight; ages 13–17 years) with formally diagnosed MDD who also reported low baseline levels of aerobic activity. All participants engaged in a 12-week exercise protocol consisting of 15 supervised exercise sessions (all participants attended all supervised sessions) and 21 independent exercise sessions (81% adherence rate, verified by actigraphy). At the end of 12 weeks (no dropouts), Children's Depression Rating Scale-Revised (CDRS-R) scores reduced from 48.9 $\pm$ 9.7 to 28.5 $\pm$ 10.4 (effect size 2.0, $P<.001$), and remission (CDRS-R <28) was achieved by 62%. These marked improvements continued to be observed at 3-month follow-up, along with increased levels of ongoing physical exercise, highlighting the plausibility of this approach for adolescents with depression, including overweight and obese adolescents.

There is 1 small well-conducted RCT that has examined the effects of physical exercise on adolescents with major depressive episodes. Hughes and colleagues[44] (Hughes CW, personal communication, 2013) examined 15 adolescents (ages 12–22 years) with formally diagnosed MDD who were randomized (single-blind) to aerobic exercise (n = 8) or to a lower-intensity stretching protocol (n = 7) for 12 weeks. At baseline, mean CDRS-R depression scores in both groups were about 53 $\pm$ 6 and mean Clinical Global Impression (CGI) score was greater than 4. Both groups improved over 12 weeks, but by week 6, the exercise group showed greater reductions in CDRS scores than the stretching group (effect size 0.35). By week 12, 100% of the participants in the exercise group met response criteria, compared with 70% of the stretchers (with response defined as CDRS-R score <28 or more >50% reduction from baseline, and CGI-I <2). Using CDRS <28 as the criterion for remission, remission at week 12 was 80% for the exercisers and 60% for the stretchers. On follow-up, both exercise groups remained in remission at 6 and 12 months, with improvements also noted in family interactions, anxiety, social involvement, and school engagement.

The findings of this RCT (and the uncontrolled study) on major depression in adolescents seem impressive. It is also impressive that youths in the RCT who engaged in stretching exercises without an aerobic protocol also showed substantial improvements. Without a placebo group, it is difficult to be certain how potent nonspecific factors may have been in contributing to these results, or whether stretching itself has antidepressant effects, but the effect size of 0.35 for aerobic exercise compared with stretching suggests a significant but not powerful effect of aerobic exercise in adolescent major depression. Participation in both aerobic or stretching exercise in the RCT produced long-lasting results across a variety of life dimensions, with improvements sustained long after the end of the protocol. The follow-up data showed that many of the participants had incorporated exercise into their routines, providing an ongoing antidepressant boost to their lives. Adherence to protocol was achieved by 90% of participants in both aerobic and stretching groups, with no dropouts, again underscoring the feasibility of adolescents with depression engaging in exercise therapy.

Adverse Effects

Adverse effects of exercise are commonly underestimated. No one would argue that these adverse effects should deter anyone from exercising, but physical exercise is hardly lacking in risks (**Box 2**). A variety of preventive measures can be taken to reduce overuse injuries in youth, including supportive supervision, modification of training regimens, stopping before excessive fatigue or exhaustion, proper equipment and other mechanical precautions, and ensuring adequate periods of rest.[45]

Mechanism of Action

Current data suggest that exercise-induced mood changes may be partially mediated by improved self-esteem, at least transiently,[46,47] and at least in some individuals. Improved self-esteem might derive from a psychological sense of improved fitness; an enhanced sense of competence, achievement, or mastery; or even satisfaction from just overcoming inertia. However, in the studies on community populations (not selected for psychiatric diagnosis), changes in mood and self-concept are sometimes correlated[36] and sometimes not.[38,48] The relationship between physical self-esteem and general self-esteem is probably subject to cultural and individual factors, without easily predictable effects on mood.

Box 2
Adverse effects of physical exercise in youth

- Running-related falls
- Fractures, ligament injuries, muscle strain, and other orthopedic injuries
- Osgood-Schlatter disease: inflammation of the tendon below the knee cap where it attaches to the tibia
- Traumatized physeal growth leading to limb deformity and limb length discrepancy
- Heat cramps, heat syncope, heat exhaustion, heat stress, and heat stroke
- Concussion
- Later osteoarthritis: wrist, knee, ankle, spine, and hip
- Sudden death: if covert cardiac condition

Other psychosocial factors may be involved in the mechanism of action of exercise on mood. Improvements in mood measures might be related to simple participation in the exercise programs, resulting from relaxation, recreation, or the release of competitive and aggressive drives. The social stimulation that accompanies group exercise may be particularly useful.

Other potential mediating factors might include exercise-induced cognitive improvements, which may lead to mood improvement (or vice versa): The findings of increased hippocampal volume and improved memory in exercising adults[49] suggest that cognitive changes should be assessed as well as mood and self-esteem changes in RCTs on exercise.

The effects of physical exercise on mood outcome in individual youths may be multilayered and related to complex physical (eg, overweight status, hippocampal volume), cultural (eg, social stimulation, race), psychological (eg, cognitive functioning, self-concept, relaxation, drive release), and perhaps diagnostic factors, in addition to the biological changes that accompany physiologic stimulation and physical fitness.

Many factors need to be examined before it can be inferred that physiologic stimulation per se is the mechanism by which physical exercise improves mood or mood disorders. The mechanisms involved in improving mood in the general population might not be the same as the mechanisms involved in improving major depression.

Sedentary Behavior

The scientific literature is making it increasingly clear that sedentary behavior operates as an independent risk factor (ie, independent of low levels of physical exercise) in contributing to a wide variety of physical and mental problems, including all-cause mortality.[47,50] Sedentary behavior includes screen-centered activity (television, computer, social media, and other electronic forms of attraction) but also includes excessive involvement in reading books, relaxing in the back yard, and doing crossword puzzles (or their more modern equivalents). The fact that sedentary behavior operates as a health risk factor independently of physical exercise means that clinicians should be attentive and responsive to this aspect of their patients' lives. Physicians' encouragement of a healthy balance of activities may turn out to be a stronger good health measure than fostering physical exercise.

Summary

In nonclinical community populations, the data on the mood benefits of exercise are mixed and still inconclusive. The effects seem real, but mild to moderate in impact (effect size 0.3–0.66). Documentation is stronger for aerobic exercise, but training for muscle strength, flexibility, and perhaps balance may also have mood benefits. A Cochrane analysis found no clear difference between low-intensity and high-intensity exercise in youth, suggesting perhaps that participation in any type of physical exercise may be approximately as helpful as specifically aerobic exercise.

For adolescents with major depressive episodes, the only 2 substantial studies, 1 uncontrolled[43] and 1 nonplacebo RCT,[44] look promising, but placebo-controlled studies are needed before any conclusions can be drawn. The estimated effect size of aerobic exercise was 0.35 compared with stretching,[44] which itself may have some antidepressant properties. More data are needed to determine whether exercise is a valid adjunctive or monotherapy for depression in youth, to examine the duration of effects of short-term exercise regimens, to assess the benefits of longer-term exercise programs, and to evaluate the potential for physical exercise to prevent relapses or more distantly future major depressive episodes. There are no systematic studies of physical exercise on preadolescents with well-diagnosed major depression and no studies on youth with bipolar depression.

Interpretation of exercise studies is complicated by concurrent interventions, patient self-selection, adherence to the exercise regimen (not only in depressed patients), and blinding issues, among other methodological issues.[51] The 2 good studies on youth with major depressive episodes showed that adherence, persistence, and high retention are possible, although many other studies found it difficult to get nonclinical youths to complete their exercise protocols in intervention programs that were probably less intensively supportive (e.g., Refs.[33,34,48]).

Despite the common belief that athletics programs in schools are important for promoting public health, schools have only small effects in enhancing overall daily activity levels,[52] and the benefit of school-based programs on children's health may be overestimated.[53] The impact may improve as research on the development of public programs, and on the varying developmental and physical needs of children within public programs, becomes more refined. The empirical questions of what intensity and type of exercise are suitable to different populations, as well as which methods are most effective for encouraging youth to expend and sustain effort on exercise, need to be clarified through empirical research.[44] Exercise is an important way of promoting children's general health,[54] so it is safe to say that physical exercise is a sensible general good health measure that can be recommended to all youths, regardless of the strength of its effects on mood or mood disorders. For psychiatric patients, physical exercise can be considered comparatively safe (despite the potential for injury), inexpensive (or potentially so), easy (or reasonably so), sensible, and, compared with other psychiatric treatments, remarkably stigma free. It is less clear whether intensive aerobic exercise is better than regular energetic walks in the park with a few friends.

BRIGHT LIGHT THERAPY AND DAWN SIMULATION

The American Psychiatric Association Task Force on CAM found that bright light (light box) therapy is effective in adults as monotherapy for seasonal depression and as adjunctive therapy for nonseasonal depression.[9] Light box therapy involves a patient sitting near an artificial bright light source with a wavelength profile intended to mimic the spectrum of sunlight, usually for about 30 minutes each morning. Initially, the rationale was that the scheduled light lengthens the photoperiod during late autumn and winter for treating seasonal affective disorder (with winter worsening), presumably by correcting the phase delay in circadian rhythms associated with depression. Some later forms of light therapy have involved altering the wavelength profile with the intent of enhancing its effectiveness.

The Task Force did not review dawn simulation, although it seems approximately equal to bright light therapy in antidepressant effectiveness for adults with seasonal affective disorder.[55] A meta-analysis in adults[56] found an effect size of 0.73 in 5 studies of dawn simulation, compared with an effect size of 0.84 in 8 studies of bright light box therapy, suggesting substantial antidepressant effects with both forms of light therapy. Dawn simulation is a different form of light therapy, in which an electronic device is attached to a regular incandescent light and controls a gradual increase in light intensity before the patient's awakening. The gradual brightening of ambient room light is typically started around 90 minutes (30–120 minutes) before the target wake-up time, beginning from light-off and slowly increasing to full bulb brightness. Light enters the eye through the closed translucent eyelids, triggering biological clocks and initiating the onset of diurnal rhythms (eg, autonomic functions, circadian hormone levels, alertness, and reaction times). This approach to light therapy is often experienced as more convenient than light boxes, because dawn simulation exerts its effects before a patient's awakening and does not require the discipline of sitting next to a light source for a fixed amount of time each day. In general, their maximum illumination level lies within the range of ordinary bright commercial incandescent light bulbs (100–300 lux, compared with 10,000 lux for light boxes). Various manufacturers are marketing these devices.

All 8 published reports on light therapy in youth have shown consistently positive effects on mood symptoms, although varying in degree. These reports focus almost exclusively on bright light (box) therapy in youths, mainly with mild to moderate depressive symptoms, in the context of various diagnoses but mostly MDD.

Three early reports on light therapy in youth were nonrandomized studies: A single case[57] of a 16-year-old with seasonal affective disorder in winter was treated with light box therapy for 1 hour each morning (intensity not reported) and showed improvement in Hamilton Depression Rating Scale (HDRS), Seasonal Affective Disorders Version score (from 32 to 7) within a week, with the effect confirmed in an ABAB (off-on-off-on) study design. An open qualitative study of 18 adolescents (ages 18–19 years) with winter seasonal affective disorder treated with light boxes (10,000 lux for 40 minutes daily)[58] found subjective improvements in ease of morning awakening and in self-reported ability to concentrate, but no improvement in observer-reported school attendance, which (in lieu of depression rating scales) was interpreted as a marker for hypersomnia and depression. In a small single-blind crossover study of light box therapy (2 hours in the evening),[59] 5 youths with winter depression (seasonal affective disorder) showed small improvements in symptoms (compared with relaxation training), but 4 youths with nonseasonal depression did not; this small study provides the only available data in youth suggesting a possible effect of seasonality as a factor affecting the effectiveness of light therapy.

The 4 RCTs on light therapy in youth[60–63] have been consistently positive, but only 2 were explicitly treating MDD.[60,61] A randomized double-blind placebo-controlled crossover study[60] examined 28 youths (ages 7–17 years) with recurrent winter MDD treated by a light therapy regimen combining dawn simulation (up to 250 lux for 2 hours in the morning) and light box therapy (2500–10,000 lux for 1 hour in the evening rather than the morning) administered for a week, and then participants were crossed over to the other treatment (half the sample received light therapy first, half received placebo first). Placebo involved sham dawn simulation (2 lux for 5 minutes) and, rather than sitting at a light box, sitting and performing a sedentary activity while wearing dark glasses for 1 hour in the evening. Using the Structured Interview Guide for the HDRS, Seasonal Affective Disorders (SIGH-SAD), children's self-ratings showed only a trend toward improvement on a depression scale ($P = .016$), but parent ratings showed a larger improvement with light therapy than placebo treatment ($P = .009$). Parent-scored rates of treatment response (defined as symptom reduction $\geq 50\%$) were 71% with light therapy compared with 25% with placebo ($P<.01$). Adverse effects were minimal and comparable in both treatments. This early report remains the most rigorous RCT on light therapy in youth with winter MDD.

A randomized placebo-controlled crossover study (blinding not mentioned) of 28 adolescents (ages 14–17 years) examined bright light box treatment as a monotherapy for nonseasonal cases of major or minor depressive disorders.[61] Entry into the study required a baseline BDI score greater than 9, and the mean baseline score of participants was 25. Bright light therapy (2500 lux) or placebo (50 lux) was administered for 1 hour daily for 1 week, then participants crossed over to the other treatment (14 received bright light therapy first, and 14 received placebo first).

Although detailed data were not provided, mean BDI scores reduced modestly from about 25 to 20 by day 7 (P = .014), with no significant adverse effects.

Bright light therapy has been examined in youth with delayed sleep-phase disorder, in which disruptions in circadian rhythm lead to a regular pattern of late bedtimes and late morning awakening times, with changes in diurnal hormonal and body temperature cycles, daily alertness (slow alerting on awakening), energy patterns, and often depressive moods,[64] typically with onset in childhood or adolescence.[65] The disorder can be transient or lifelong, and melatonin can be helpful to a degree.[66] In the 1 RCT examining bright light therapy to treat delayed sleep-phase disorder in youth,[62] 49 adolescents (ages 11–18 years) with delayed sleep-phase disorder (mean duration over 4 years, 16% having school absenteeism) were randomized to receive bright light therapy plus cognitive-behavioral therapy (n = 26) or to a waiting list (n = 23). The treated adolescents received morning bright light therapy (1000 lux or sunlight for 30–120 minutes) combined with cognitive-behavioral therapy (6 45-minute to 60-minute sessions of sleep hygiene education and cognitive restructuring of sleep-related cognitions). After 8 weeks, the treated adolescents showed a reduction in depression scores (on the Short Mood and Feelings Questionnaire, which is not confounded by sleep items) from 7.6 ± 3.6 to 3.9 ± 2.8 (effect size d = 0.71 compared with controls), along with improvements in sleep onset (d = 0.65–1.13), bedtime (d = 0.89–1.24), awakening time (d = 0.92), daytime sleepiness (d = 0.79), and fatigue (d = 0.75). After treatment, diagnostic criteria for delayed sleep-phase disorder were met by fewer treated than untreated adolescents (13% vs 82%, P<.0001). Most improvements persisted at 6-month follow-up (depression scores d = 0.86, P = .01). Although the number of study participants who met criteria of MDD was not specified, this result is an impressive improvement in both mood and sleep items in a sleep disorder that is difficult to treat and that often clinically mimics MDD.

One case report and 1 RCT have examined the effects of bright light therapy on mood in youths with eating disorders. The case report[67] described a 17-year-old with a restrictive eating disorder not otherwise specified presenting with winter exacerbations of her eating and mood symptoms. Although the report did not cite a mood diagnosis, the clinical description suggested a probable seasonal MDD. Morning bright light therapy (10,000 lux for 30 minutes) seemed to produce some clinical improvement in eating and mood symptoms after 4 days. After 1 month of treatment, improvement was observed in depression scores (BDI scores reduced from 37 to 17, SIGH-SAD from 12 to 3) and in eating symptoms and medical status, with continued improvement over the subsequent months. The RCT study[63] examined 24 girls (ages 15–20 years) with anorexia nervosa-restrictive type and depressive symptoms (HDRS ≥17), but there was no mention of whether any participants had MDD or seasonality. The patients, who received cognitive-behavioral therapy throughout the study, were randomly assigned to receive either bright light treatment (n = 12, 10,000 lux for 30 minutes daily) or no additional treatment apart from cognitive-behavioral therapy (n = 12). There was no placebo group. Depression ratings improved in both treatment groups, but were significantly more improved in the light therapy group (relative to the control group) after 5 weeks (P<0.02). Remission (HDRS ≤8) at 6 weeks was achieved by more of the adolescents treated with bright light therapy (75% vs 8%). Body mass index was beginning to improve as well, but it had not reached significance (relative to the control group) at 6 weeks. Neither of the 2 studies on eating disorders reported on possible mood diagnoses, so it is unclear whether bright light therapy had a direct effect on the eating disorder symptoms or an indirect effect mediated through improvement in comorbid mood disorders. Although the data regarding eating disorders in youth remain sparse, both reports appeared to show beneficial effects, so the benign nature of bright light therapy renders it a defensible adjunctive measure for treating youth with eating disorders,[68] and especially in cases with comorbid depression.

Adverse effects of light box therapy are generally mild (**Box 3**), but the inconvenience of the treatment is considerable, with a 19% discontinuation rate in adults[69] and probably a higher rate in youth. Significant adverse effects of dawn simulation are rarely reported. Mania associated with light therapy has been reported in adults,[70–73] but apparently not yet in youth.

Summary

Although the role of publication bias in producing these consistently positive findings cannot be excluded, the 4 open-label reports (total n = 25) and 4 RCTs (total n = 129) on light therapy all showed positive effects on mood or mood disorders in youth. The available data have mainly examined adolescents using bright light box therapy, typically with mild to moderate depressive symptoms or disorders. The effects seem to be mostly substantial, often appearing within 1 week and consistently by 4 to 6 weeks. The available data do not permit an easy estimate of overall response rate or effect size in youth, but taken as a group, the findings seem to provide fair support for the effectiveness of bright light therapy for treating depressive moods in youth. The best RCT on winter seasonal affective disorder found that light therapy (combining light box and dawn simulation) produced substantial symptom improvement in 71% of the sample, compared with 25% on placebo.[60] The best RCT on nonseasonal depression[61] found a weaker effect. The RCT on delayed sleep-phase disorder[62] showed a strong benefit, so light therapies for treating this depression-like condition should be pursued in further research, in addition to studies on actual mood disorders.

Although bright light therapy seems to be effective in adults as a monotherapy for seasonal depression and as an adjunctive therapy for nonseasonal depression, better data in youth are needed to assess the role of seasonality, the effectiveness of adjunctive therapy versus monotherapy, its value for severe depression versus mild to moderate depression, and its effects in bipolar disorder. Dawn simulation should be receiving more research attention in general, but especially in children. There is a need for adequately powered RCTs in children and adolescents comparing light box therapy, dawn simulation, and some of the newer technologies using specific wavelength profiles.

Although its adverse effects are minimal for an antidepressant treatment, light box therapy is time-consuming and inconvenient. It can be a demanding procedure for children and may be unfeasible for some. The devices are not covered by most insurance plans ($100–$500), but some third-party payers are starting to provide

---

Box 3
Adverse effects of bright light box therapy

- Eye strain or irritation
- Vision changes
- Headache
- Nausea or abdominal discomfort
- Autonomic hyperstimulation
- Insomnia
- Mania

reimbursement. The initial presumption that light box therapy is effective because it extends the photoperiod is challenged by the strong data suggesting that it is also a helpful adjunctive treatment of nonseasonal MDD in adults, a finding that raises questions about the simple assumptions linking mood and circadian rhythms in general, and broadens the range of potential indications worthy of study. There are anecdotal suggestions that light therapy is helpful for mood and alertnesss in people who are not clinically depressed, and this does not seem to have been systematically investigated. Dawn simulation is especially worth investigating for youth, who may be unable to manage the self-discipline required for light box therapy. It is remarkable that a reasonably safe, inexpensive, biologically sensible treatment that has been so well established in adults has received so little systematic study in youth.

ST. JOHN'S WORT (HYPERICUM)

Hypericum, a herb used for centuries to treat depression, is an invasive weed that can be made into an extract that is delivered in liquid or pill form. The extracts can be made from the leaf, flower, or fruit, and they contain various chemical constituents, depending on the plant genetics, soil, weather and seasonal effects, harvesting techniques, mixture of plant components, and extraction methods. Its various and varied chemical ingredients have differing pharmacologic effects on serotonin, norepinephrine, dopamine, and other neurotransmitters, in addition to its neuroendocrinologic and neuroimmunologic properties.[74] Although it might be considered an advantage that hypericum can enhance the effects of 3 different neurotransmitter systems, this property could also be viewed as a disadvantage, in that unnecessary neuronal pathways may be variably stimulated. The governmentally unregulated commercial extracts of St. John's wort in the United States are known to contain highly varied amounts of the main active ingredients in hypericum. High batch-to-batch variability in the amounts of hyperforin and hypericin (the main active ingredients of hypericum) complicates the reproducibility and reliability of its effects, even within the product of a single brand.[75] These extracts also contain a variety of other neurochemically active agents with poorly characterized properties. For clinical use, hypericum might be considered a pharmacologically dirty antidepressant compared with single-agent pharmaceuticals.

In adults, numerous meta-analyses suggest that hypericum is equal in efficacy to conventional antidepressants for treating mild to moderate depression, reportedly with fewer adverse effects.[9,76,77] The CAM Task Force of the American Psychiatric Association concluded that hypericum monotherapy "may be a reasonable treatment for mild to moderate MDD."[9] This language falls short of endorsing hypericum as efficacious. Furthermore, the value of St. John's wort is less clear for adults with severe MDD.

In youth, there are only 3 studies, and all are open-label. In a 4-week to 6-week open-label study of a hypericum extract containing 300 to 1800 mg daily (standardized as equivalent to 0.9–7.2 mg of hypericin), 101 children (ages ≤12 years) with mild to moderate depressive symptoms (but not MDD) were described by physicians' impressions rather than rating scales, so there was no statistical analysis.[78] Physicians reported good or excellent improvement in 72% of the sample after 2 weeks and in 97% of the children who completed the 4-week to 6-week study; however, 25% of the sample had dropped out. These are impressive results and impressively rapid changes, but the informal study design renders these findings as suggestive at best.

A more rigorous open-label study by Findling[79] examined 33 youths (ages 6–16 years) with moderate or severe MDD (CDRS-R ≥40, CGI ≥4) using a hypericum extract 150 to 300 mg 3 times daily. At baseline, CDRS scores were 56 ± 8, and CGI-Severity scores were 4.2 ± 0.6. Significant improvement in CDRS-R depression scores and global improvement (CGI) scores were noted at 1 week (P<.01). Response criteria (CDRS-R ≤28 and CGI-Severity ≤2) were met by 24% of the intent-to-treat sample at 4 weeks and by 83% at 8 weeks. Dropout rate was 9%. Of the 8-week completers, 93% elected to continue treatment with hypericum after the trial ended. Adverse effects were mild and transient (dizziness, increased appetite, or loose stools), with no weight gain, laboratory abnormalities, or electrocardiogram (EKG) changes. A dose of 900 mg daily, which is a typical adult dose, was tolerated by 57% of children and 83% of adolescents. This well-conducted open-label study suggests that hypericum might have a strong antidepressant effect in youth with MDD, including a rapid response at 1 week.

The third open-label study by Simeon,[80] examining hypericum extract 300 mg 3 times daily in 33 adolescents (ages 12–17 years) with mild to moderate MDD (baseline CDRS 40.9 ± 11.5), also reported significant improvements after just 1 week of treatment: BDI (P = .003), CGI (P = .002), CDRS (P = .0001), and Montgomery-Asberg Depression Rating Scale (P = .008). Of the 11 adolescents who completed the 8-week study, 9 youths (82%) were scored as "much improved" or "very much improved" on the CGI at 8 weeks. However, there was a 57% dropout rate, so only 9 of 26 (35%) improved on intent-to-treatment analysis based on CGI scores at 8 weeks. Also, perhaps because of the more aggressive dosing strategy, a high incidence of adverse effects was reported in this study (with 35%–40% reporting restlessness, dry mouth, nightmares, confusion, and inattention), but again no weight, laboratory, or EKG changes. Nonetheless, for completers, this open-label study showed substantial improvements, which again were observable in 1 week.

In addition to the 3 open-label clinical trials, there is a manufacturer's postmarketing surveillance study in Germany on 101 children (ages 1 to 12 years, median 9 years) who were treated for 4 to 6 weeks with a hypericum extract of 300 to 1800 mg (standardized to a hypericin dose of 0.9–5.4 mg) daily.[78] Unvalidated qualitative questionnaires were completed by physicians and parents to assess therapeutic and adverse effects. Physicians rated overall clinical responses as good or excellent in 72% at 2 weeks and 100% at 6 weeks, and parent ratings were 65% and 98%. However, 9% of the sample had dropped out by week 4, and 24% of the initial sample failed to provide any data at week 6. Symptoms suggestive of depression (but not items used in the Diagnostic and Statistical Manual of Mental Disorders) were rated and also showed unlikely and inflated suggestions of improvement, and no adverse effects were reported. This study does not seem to provide reliable clinical information.

Hypericum has been widely used in Germany, where it is a government-approved treatment of depression, but its use in youth seems to have been decreasing dramatically in recent years. A rigorous study estimated that hypericum accounted for 56% of antidepressant use in German youth in the year 2000,[81] whereas data from a health insurance company found that only 8.5% of adolescents were prescribed hypericum in 2009.[82] Although the difference in methodologies used to make these estimates may misrepresent the extent of the shift, this seeming change in usage patterns suggests an increasing compliance by clinicians with guideline recommendations to use selective serotonin reuptake inhibitors (SSRIs) as first-line treatments for depression.[82] It also suggests an increasing sense by German physicians of the clinical limitations of hypericum.

Adverse effects of hypericum include side effects typical of serotonin reuptake inhibitors (SRIs), including sexual side effects and discontinuation syndrome (**Box 4**). In adults, the serotonergic side effects of hypericum may be fewer than with SSRIs.[77,83] An unconfirmed report in an adult[84] suggests that hypericum might have antithyroid effects, denoted by an increase in thyroid-stimulating hormone (TSH) levels, but this possibility has been questioned on physiologic grounds.[85] Favorable features of its side effect profile include the absence of effects on weight, blood pressure, EKG, or other laboratory tests.

Questions have been raised about whether hypericum might induce seizures. The data from MedWatch system for voluntary reporting of adverse clinical effects to the US Food and Drug Administration (FDA) are ambiguous.[86] Animal models give evidence of both anticonvulsant[87–89] and proconvulsant properties,[87,90] perhaps consistent with the highly variable contents of hypericum extracts. A case report[91] describes seizures apparently induced by a hypericum overdose in a 16-year-old who was self-treating depression with over-the-counter St. John's wort in huge quantities; she ingested up to 15 pills (300 mg each) daily for 2 weeks and then 50 pills in a possible suicide attempt just before a generalized seizure (diffuse spike and wave electroencephalographic [EEG] pattern). Although the literature on hypericum does not directly support a risk of seizures except in overdose, it is reasonable to extend the FDA Black Box warnings of 2004 and 2007 about the seizure-inducing potential of all commercial antidepressants[92,93] to include hypericum as well. Its use in patients with epilepsy should be approached cautiously, especially in view of possible drug interactions with anticonvulsant agents.

Drug interactions are significant for hypericum, which induces the cytochrome P450 isozymes CYP3A4, 2C19, and 2C9 as well as the *P*-glycoprotein transporter.[94] As an example relevant to adolescent females, more rapid clearance of estradiol may reduce the effectiveness of oral contraception. Because of the risks of serotonin syndrome, it is sensible to ask all patients receiving psychiatric medications about their possible unreported use of hypericum. One report[95] described 5 youths who used hypericum

---

Box 4
Adverse effects of hypericum (St. John's wort)

- Increased or decreased appetite, diarrhea, constipation, nausea, dyspepsia
- Dizziness, headache, impaired attention, confusion
- Insomnia, vivid dreams, nightmares
- Restlessness, anxiety, irritability, agitation, mania
- SSRI effects, including sexual side effects, serotonin syndrome, discontinuation syndrome
- Sedation or fatigue
- Dry mouth
- Sexual side effects
- Photosensitivity
- Increased TSH levels: questionable
- No changes in weight, blood pressure, EKG, or other laboratory tests
- Note drug interactions: induction of cytochromes P450 3A4, 2C19, and 2C9 and the P-glycoprotein transporter.

without informing their psychopharmacologists. Intolerance of low doses of other psychiatric or general medical drugs should also raise concern about possible covert use of hypericum.

Clinical Note

Despite the minimal data in youth, some clinicians may consider hypericum for patients who strongly prefer nonpharmaceutical treatments, who have failed on multiple conventional antidepressants, or who lack insurance and have limited financial resources to support conventional treatment. Hypericum is commercially available as St. John's wort extracts, which are typically standardized to be equivalent to 0.125% to 0.3% hypericin or 3% to 5% hyperforin. Using 300 mg to 900 mg capsules (containing 0.3% hypericin), a standard starting dose in adults is 300 mg 3 times daily (or 450 mg twice daily), increasing as tolerated to 600 mg 3 times daily. In children, a starting dose might be 150 mg 3 times daily, with increases up to 300 mg or 600 mg 3 times daily, although some children may tolerate only 150 mg daily. Some clinical improvement may be seen in 1 to 2 weeks, but the main clinical response comes in 2 to 8 weeks, similar to the time lag with pharmaceutical antidepressants. After a period of stabilization, a maintenance dose at 75% (down to 25%) of full dosage might be sufficient. Brands that might be considered include Nature's Way, Soloray, Source Natural, Thorne, or Pure Encapsulations. The 2013 cost is about $1 to $2 daily for a 900-mg to 1800-mg dose.

Summary

In all 3 open-label reports in youth with MDD, impressive clinical changes were noted after only 1 to 2 weeks of treatment, with reasonably strong improvement seen in some youths. Two of the studies had high dropout rates (25%–57%), limiting the overall response rate at 4 to 8 weeks to a modest level; the third study had a low dropout rate (9%) and showed substantial responses. Drug interactions with hypericum are a prominent concern, given its induction of some drug-metabolizing cytochromes that may reduce the effectiveness of a variety of medications, including birth control pills. Physicians need to be wary of unreported home usage of hypericum in combination with conventional antidepressant treatments, which can elicit serotonin syndrome and other unexpected adverse effects. Lack of product standardization of unregulated herbal extracts is a problem, adding another layer of unpredictability: The effectiveness of 1 brand of hypericum cannot be generalized to imply the effectiveness of other brands.[77] Although sticking with 1 preferred effective brand can help, clinicians need to be mindful of batch-to-batch variability.[75] Physicians should bear in mind that the evidence in adults suggests that hypericum may be more useful in mild to moderate MDD than in severe cases, although the preliminary open-label data in youth suggest that it might be helpful across the full range of severity.

There are no controlled studies of hypericum in youth, but the mixed findings in the 3 small open trials are encouraging enough to warrant proper RCTs. However, in view of the known complications and unpredictabilities of hypericum, most physicians will probably prefer to use other antidepressant agents. Even if hypericum were shown to have antidepressant efficacy in youth, its main clinical value might be for patients or families who cannot reconcile themselves to the use of pharmaceuticals. However, its main strength is low cost, which may be a deciding factor in some clinical situations.

S-ADENOSYLMETHIONINE

This ubiquitous and multipotent molecule is involved in thousands of biological reactions across wide expanses of general metabolism (methylation, sulfuration, alkylation, aminopropylation) and is essential to epigenetic processes (SAMe is the main methyl donor for DNA methylation).[96] As a small part of its domain, SAMe exerts a broad range of neuropharmacologic effects[97,98] beyond the synthesis of serotonin, dopamine, and norepinephrine. Early studies over several decades showed little or no antidepressant effectiveness, probably because the older commercial synthetic processes were inefficient, and the hygroscopic properties of SAMe (readily breaking down when exposed to water) rendered the ingredients inactive. SAMe remains a difficult substance to synthesize properly, and some consumer groups have found that commercial products labeled as SAMe on drugstore shelves may contain no detectable SAMe. More recent research studies have used higher-grade SAMe. The CAM Task Force of the American Psychiatric Association has determined that SAMe is efficacious as monotherapy for adults with MDD when used in the range of 400 to 1600 mg daily.[9]

Despite this strong endorsement for treating MDD in adults, there is only 1 open-label report on 3 youths (ages 8–16 years) with clinically diagnosed MDD.[99] When treated with 600 to 1400 mg daily, similar to the adult dose range, all 3 youths showed a rapid treatment response (CDI scores were reported in 2 patients, with a mean reduction from 31 to 5) within 1 to 2 weeks. Benefits persisted throughout a 22-week follow-up period. One patient, whose therapeutic response was confirmed in a naturalistic ABAB reversal (off-on-off-on), noted mild anxiety and tremor, which were relieved at a lower dose.

Adverse effects are generally minimal. Clinicians should monitor for the expectable side effects associated with the psychostimulant and tricyclic antidepressant properties of SAMe, including mania and possible serotonin syndrome (**Box 5**). Anxiety does seem to increase in many youths, especially if there were previous anxiety symptoms. Despite strong warnings about mania in the lay literature, SAMe is probably no more (or less) likely than other antidepressants to induce mania, and routine monitoring precautions are advisable. There is 1 reported adult case of a suicide attempt shortly after starting SAMe treatment.[100] There have been no reports of weight gain, sexual side effects, seizures, or changes in laboratory tests or EKG with SAMe.

Summary

Despite the potential advantages of its adverse effect profile, the use of SAMe in adults with MDD has never been widely adopted by psychiatrists, perhaps

---

Box 5
Adverse effects of SAMe

- Anxiety, insomnia, agitation, mania
- Tricyclic antidepressant effects, including sexual side effects, discontinuation syndrome, serotonin syndrome (rare), and mania
- Psychostimulant side effects, including anxiety, anorexia, insomnia, tachycardia, sweating, tremor, headache, and dizziness
- Dyspepsia, anorexia, nausea/vomiting, diarrhea, constipation, flatulence
- Homocysteinemia: questionable
- No changes in weight, sexual side effects, seizures, EKG, or other laboratory tests

because this natural antidepressant cannot be patented by pharmaceutical houses. With low profits for the pharmaceutical industry, SAMe lacks the visibility in journal advertising and marketing campaigns that would allow it to rival other efficacious antidepressants. This situation highlights the critical role that pharmaceutical advertising plays in physicians' choice of treatments, and it showcases the disadvantage that effective CAM treatments have in real-world competition with extensively marketed agents in gaining a foothold in the treatment armamentarium. It is a sad comment that, despite the numerous RCTs showing efficacy in adults, insurance companies do not reimburse for this inexpensive treatment ($1–$4 daily).

There is a similar situation pertaining to the potential use of SAMe for treating youth with attention-deficit hyperactivity disorder (ADHD), with or without depression. Shekim and colleagues[101] conducted a small RCT in adults in 1990, showing that 6 of 8 adults with ADHD showed moderate to marked improvement. In youth, the only available study on SAMe in ADHD is a small randomized double-blind placebo-controlled trial involving 7 participants with ADHD and 22q11.2 chromosome deletion syndrome,[102] which is often called velocardiofacial syndrome in psychiatry. In addition to congenital physical abnormalities, multisystem medical complications, cognitive deficits, speech and language impairments, and a variety of psychiatric symptoms,[103] about 30% of these children fulfill criteria for ADHD,[104] which is partially responsive to methylphenidate.[105] The 7 youths (ages 9–15 years) with this deletion syndrome showed no improvement in ADHD Rating Scale-IV scores or on cognitive measures[106] with SAMe doses up to 800 mg twice daily (mean not specified) for 6 weeks. The negative findings in this study are tempered by the medical complexities in this population and the limited number of participants. In view of the positive findings in the small RCT in adults and encouraging anecdotal clinical observations in youth with ADHD, it is remarkable that there are no RCTs on SAMe for treating ADHD in medically healthy youth or adults.

This effective and established (if rarely used) treatment in adults has been examined in only 1 small open-label trial in youth with depression, so studies are sorely needed. In my own clinical practice, SAMe seems to be a helpful monotherapy (or carefully titrated adjunctive therapy) for children and adolescents with MDD or ADHD, especially in the absence of prominent symptoms of anxiety.

Clinical Note
___

Despite the minimal data in youth, some clinical circumstances might lead practitioners to consider the use of SAMe. Because of the difficulties in the commercial synthesis of SAMe, patients should be directed to carefully selected brands, and because hygroscopicity limits its shelf-life, supplies should be kept new, dry, and cool. Reliable brands, including Nature Made, Jarrow, and Natrol, make 200-mg and 400-mg enteric-coated pills, which are preferably taken on an empty stomach. Similar to psychostimulants, the primary dose is administered in the morning, but additional doses may be added during the day. The starting dose is 200 mg, and increases of 200-mg steps may proceed every 5 to 10 days, with a typical full dose in children of 400 to 800 mg (compared with 400–1600 mg in adults), although higher doses may be used if tolerated. Maximal dose is often limited by an increase in anxiety. Some partial improvement may appear in 1 to 2 weeks, but the usual time lag is 2 to 8 weeks for the full antidepressant effect. (The anti-ADHD effect may be evident within days.) The 2013 cost is about $1.50 to $3.00 daily for an 800-mg dose.

5-HYDROXYTRYPTOPHAN

The CAM Task Force of the American Psychiatric Association did not report on 5-hydroxytryptophan (5HTP) because of a paucity of data.[9] An older Cochrane review on adults with MDD in 2002 found that only 2 of 27 RCTs on either tryptophan or 5HTP had adequate methodology, although those 2 RCTs showed substantial and rapid benefit.[107,108] Based on those 2 studies in adults, the Cochrane report viewed the data as suggesting that 5HTP was better than placebo (OR 4.1, number needed to treat [NNT] 2.8), with a clinical response observable in 3 to 7 days; however, it drew no conclusion because of insufficient data and emphasized that additional studies were needed on both efficacy and safety, especially in view of the fatalities associated with the eosinophilia-myalgia syndrome.

Eosinophilia-Myalgia Syndrome

Clinical psychiatric research on 5HTP virtually halted 20 years ago in response to the emergence of eosinophilia-myalgia syndrome. A large number of serious cases (at least 1500 cases, at least 37 deaths) of this sclerodermalike condition were eventually attributed to a faulty manufacturing process of tryptophan by a single company in a foreign country. A series of manufacturing violations were uncovered in the late 1980s at this particular manufacturing plant, several of which may have contributed to the defective tryptophan products. Some 5HTP batches were found to be problematic as well,[109–111] and the FDA banned both products in 1991. The key fact about this historically important scare is that there have been no new cases since 1992.[112,113] There is a possible exception in the case of an adult in 2009 who used L-tryptophan in combination with some other agents after duodenal-switch weight loss surgery[114]; this isolated case suggests that there might be rare idiosyncratic occurrences of this syndrome, which is in fact known to be associated with other causes.[115] Since the lifting of the FDA ban in 2002, the FDA has blocked the importation of foreign-sourced tryptophan and 5HTP, and the FDA now oversees the manufacturing of these products in the United States. A historically pivotal effect of the scare is that it has dramatically delayed clinical investigation of this unpatentable compound, and research on its use in depression is now overdue to restart in both adults and youth. Little additional clinical data on 5HTP in adults with depression have accumulated in the intervening years.

CLINICAL USE OF 5HTP

In adults, early studies from the 1970's and 1980's showed mixed effects of 5HTP in treating depression in adults, but these were all open-label and brief (less than 4 weeks) trials in treatment-resistant cases.[116–119] In youth, there are no open-label reports at all on 5HTP for depression, but some clinical and research reports have examined it in youth for other purposes. An early report on 2 children (ages 7 and 9 years) with probable autism showed no observable changes that were attributable to 5HTP at a dose of 3 mg/kg.[120] Another early report of 3 children (ages 4–8 years) with severe autism (and mean IQ 52) examined in a fixed-sequence (ABA) double-blind placebo-controlled study of 5HTP (300–500 mg daily with carbidopa 100 mg) also found no behavioral improvements,[121] although agitation was noted at these high doses; no standardized mood measure was used, but observer-rated smiling showed no consistent changes. Assessment of mood in these children would have been difficult at best, but neither report identified any mood effect. Several reports on 5HTP treatment in children with migraine[122–124] or Lesch-Nyhan syndrome[125–129] either found no mood effects or did not assess mood effects. Regarding sleep disorders, a double-blind pla-cebo-controlled crossover study of 48 students with headaches and sleep disorders found improvements in headaches, frequent awakenings, and some parasomnias.[130] In an open-label study of children (ages 3–11 years) with night terrors (pavor noctur-nus), 31 children were treated with 5HTP (2 mg/kg nightly) and compared with 14 chil-dren who received no treatment; after 1 month, improvement was observed in 93% of treated and 29% of untreated children, and after 6 months of treatment, 84% of treated youths were free of sleep terrors compared with 39% of the untreated youths.[131] These studies do not provide data regarding effects on mood in youth, but the last 2 small trials suggest the feasibility of 5HTP treatment in youth and its po-tential to enhance sleep.

In addition to these clinical reports, several psychiatric research reports in children have used a 5HTP infusion test as a biological marker to assess serotonergic func-tioning,[132–134] but these acute studies did not assess effects on mood. There are no useful data on 5HTP effects on mood or mood disorders in youth. Nonetheless, despite the gap in research on 5HTP in psychiatry, its potential deserves serious consideration.

Physiologic Chemistry of 5HTP

5HTP is a unique natural candidate as a treatment of depression: 5HTP is the imme-diate precursor molecule to serotonin and is converted to serotonin by a single enzyme. In a pathway relevant to depressive disorders, once the amino acid trypto-phan is hydroxylated to 5HTP, the enzyme L-aromatic amino acid decarboxylase converts 5HTP to serotonin. (Similarly, in the pathway relevant to Parkinson disease, after the amino acid tyrosine is converted to L-dopa, this same decarboxylase converts L-dopa to dopamine.) The clinical advantage of using 5HTP rather than tryp-tophan is that tryptophan is largely diverted in the body to protein formation and other metabolic functions, whereas 5HTP is primarily metabolized to serotonin. Because only small amounts of 5HTP are diverted to other biochemical pathways (specifically toward kyurenine), most of the 5HTP that is present in the brain is converted to sero-tonin and is thereby able to exert a highly selective influence on serotoninergic receptors.

Even more than the cleanest of the SSRIs, 5HTP is uniquely able to stimulate enhance serotonin neurotransmission without stimulating other neuroreceptors or collateral pathways. With fewer side effects resulting from collateral pathways, 5HTP doses can be increased to attain a stronger serotonergic stimulation. 5HTP is cleaner and more selectively serotonergic than the most selective of the SSRIs, and it provides the strongest serotonergic stimulation currently available.

Carbidopa in Combination with 5HTP

The enhancement of 5HTP by carbidopa allows for an even stronger and cleaner 5HTP effect. Carbidopa is a prescription medication commonly used in combination with L-dopa to enhance its treatment of Parkinson disease. Carbidopa, which does not readily cross the blood-brain barrier, has the capacity to strongly inhibit the L-aromatic amino acid decarboxylase enzyme outside the brain. In Parkinsons disease, its use blocks the peripheral conversion of L-dopa to dopamine, thereby reducing the peripheral side effects of dopamine on the cardiovascular and gastroin-testinal systems (hypotension, arrhythmias, nausea, gastrointestinal bleeding), and simultaneously increasing the availability of L-dopa for entry into the brain. Similarly, the use of carbidopa with 5HTP reduces the peripheral formation of serotonin and its attendant peripheral cardiac and gastrointestinal side effects, and concurrently increasing the plasma 5HTP levels by 5-fold to 15-fold[135,136] and enhancing 5HTP delivery to the brain. Carbidopa provides for stronger central effects of 5HTP with few peripheral effects.[137–139] It also allows the use of lower oral doses of 5HTP, although many of the early studies of 5HTP in treating depression in adults used high doses of 5HTP in combination with carbidopa or other decarboxylase inhibitors (eg, Refs.[137,140–144]).

Although there are no data on the 5HTP/carbidopa combination for treating depression in youth, the 3 clinical studies in children have used 5HTP doses in the range of 100 to 500 mg daily in combination with carbidopa,[121,124,127] and child psychiatric research studies evaluating serotonergic functioning in youth have used also this combination approach.[132–134]

Adverse Effects

5HTP is generally well tolerated in adults, although some adverse effects have been reported,[144] mainly consisting of transient gastrointestinal effects and the expectable treatment-emergent effects directly tied to serotonergic stimulation (**Box 6**). These treatment-emergent effects (ie, adverse effects that are directly and unavoidably tied to serotonin neurotransmission rather than stimulation of collateral pathways) are all well-known effects of SSRI treatment, and they include feelings of stomach fullness early in meals, frontal apathy or behavioral disinhibition (because of serotonin effects on frontal lobe functioning[145–147]), serotonin syndrome, and mania. 5HTP taken at bedtime is often an effective sleep aid, but excessive doses can produce a mania-like interference with sleep. Although 5HTP has anxiety-reducing therapeutic benefits,

---

Box 6
Adverse effects of 5HTP

- Sedation, but insomnia is possible at excessive doses
- Mania, agitation, or behavioral excitation
- Anxiety, tremor, headache
- Weird dreams or nightmares, especially with excessive doses taken at bedtime or for 1–5 days after dose increases
- Apathy or behavioral disinhibition at excessive doses (frontal lobe)
- Feelings of stomach fullness earlier in meals
- Nausea, vomiting, heartburn, dyspepsia, diarrhea, flatulence (reduced by concurrent use of carbidopa)
- Possible sexual side effects (infrequently reported)
- Palpitations (preventable with carbidopa)
- Serotonin syndrome at high doses or if combined with serotonergic drugs
- Possible discontinuation syndrome (infrequently reported)
- Occasional increased tendency toward bleeding
- Eosinophilia-myalgia syndrome: see text
- No weight gain, seizures, or suicidality (as yet reported)

Note: drug interactions with all serotonergic agents.

it can aggravate anxiety in some cases. In adults, gastrointestinal side effects and palpitations have been reported, but these peripheral serotonergic effects can be markedly reduced and possibly eliminated by using 5HTP in combination with carbidopa. A patient with a mitochondrial encephalomyopathy developed status epilepticus during 5HTP treatment.[148] I am unaware of any documented cases of suicidality associated with the use of 5HTP in adults or youth.

Regarding carbidopa, virtually all of the available data on adverse effects of carbidopa were obtained in adults who were also on L-dopa, and their side effects appeared to be characteristic side effects of L-dopa. Carbidopa monotherapy (without 5HTP) has been examined in youth with other medical conditions without evidence of significant adverse effects.[149,150] Carbidopa seems to have minimal if any known adverse effects of its own and does not present drug interaction issues, apart from with L-dopa or 5HTP. (Although carbidopa does not seem to have drug interactions, 5HTP does interact with all serotonergic agents.)

Medical Monitoring of 5HTP

In the absence of systematic clinical studies of 5HTP, medical monitoring should be vigilant. If clinical treatment with 5HTP is undertaken, several precautions should be considered. Both 5HTP and carbidopa can independently increase prolactin levels.[151] 5HTP combined with carbidopa can increase cortisol and prolactin levels in youth and adults.[132,133,136,152,153] Periodic monitoring of prolactin is advisable, and monitoring cortisol should be considered. In addition, liver and kidney function tests could be monitored, although more based on general principles than on specific concerns. This treatment might be contraindicated for cardiac patients, especially if there are palpitations or if the clinical condition is unstable; however, concurrent use of carbidopa should minimize cardiac effects, although EKG monitoring would still be advised.

Author's Personal Opinion

Emphasizing again that the literature does not provide systematic effectiveness or safety data for this treatment in youth, my clinical experience suggests that 5HTP can be helpful in treating children and adolescents (and adults) with MDD. Especially when combined with carbidopa to reduce its peripheral side effects and increase its central effects, 5HTP seems often able to help treatment-resistant depression in patients who have had unsuccessful trials of 2 or more SSRIs. An added benefit is that proper dosing of 5HTP+carbidopa often has noticeably fewer adverse effects than SRIs. In addition to treating depression and treatment-resistant depression, I find that 5HTP+carbidopa can be useful for treating anxiety disorders, obsessive compulsive disorder, insomnia, and carbohydrate craving. Because of its apparent (although putative) antidepressant effects and generally minimal adverse effects, I have used it as a first-line treatment of depression, often in preference to SSRIs (although exclusively in cases in which the patient and/or family understand the significance of considering an alternative treatment without available controlled trials before trying established treatments, and only in those cases in which informed consent can be considered genuinely valid and is carefully documented in the patient's record, and only when the clinical acuity and severity of the patient are mild enough to allow departing from standard treatment).

Rigorous clinical trials are needed before this treatment can be recommended, but some guidance is offered for researchers and for the rare clinical situations in which this approach might be valid. When 5HTP is used without carbidopa, the typical dose range for treating depression is 50 to 300 or even 600 mg daily in adults. 5HTP is available over-the-counter in 50-mg, 10-mg, or 200-mg pills. Effective brands include Jarrow, Natrol, Solgar, and Nature's Bounty. The 2013 cost is about $1 daily for a 200-mg to 400-mg dose (about $2.50 daily if used with carbidopa). Many people are able to use over-the-counter 5HTP without difficulty, although they may have a few adverse gastrointestinal or other side effects.

When using 5HTP with carbidopa, I suggest starting 5HTP with dramatically lower doses, even although high doses were used in short-term infusion studies or single-dose challenge tests in a research setting. I typically recommend that youths (and adults) begin carbidopa with 25 mg each morning for 2 days, then 50 mg each morning for 2 days. (A typical adult dose for carbidopa is 75 to 200 mg daily, although studies have suggested that doses up to 300–450 mg are safe,[149,153,154] so the 50 mg daily dose recommended here seems modest.) After the 4-day carbidopa lead-in, I usually recommend starting with 1 or 2 mg of 5HTP in the morning, preferably with carbohydrates, and then working up gradually (1–2 mg every 3–7 days) from that dose. Because 50 mg is the smallest available commercial dose, it is necessary to enlist a compounding pharmacy to prepare capsules containing 1 mg of 5HTP (advising the pharmacist to obtain a high-grade manufacturer's product.) Most children and adolescents taking carbidopa achieve a final dose of 5HTP in the range of 5 to 15 mg (occasionally up to 25 mg, or 50 mg in adults). Higher doses of 5HTP, even when combined with carbidopa, have been used in some adult[144] and child[121] studies, but may not be necessary. Larger 5HTP pills can be compounded for patients needing higher doses. For the small number of patients who find 1 mg daily to be too high, the starting dose can be reduced to 0.1 mg (or sometimes 0.01 mg), and then increased gradually from there. If the patient has sleep symptoms, a portion of the 5HTP can be moved to nighttime. Typical onset of sedative effects is seen in 30 to 45 minutes, but sedation with daytime usage seems minimal for most patients (or doses can be temporarily decreased or moved to bedtime). In my opinion, the typical onset of the antidepressant effect is about 2 to 8 weeks, comparable with conventional antidepressants.

If carbidopa is used in combination with 5HTP, 2 clinical caveats should be emphasized. When carbidopa is prescribed for treating Parkinsons disease, it is typically combined in a pill with L-dopa (eg, Sinemet). Some pharmacists, when presented with a prescription for carbidopa, may inappropriately dispense a combination drug like Sinemet. For this reason, it is sensible to take the precaution of writing "Not Sinemet" on the prescription to reduce confusion and potential risk. Another approach is to write the prescription for Lodosyn, the only available commercial product containing carbidopa alone; it is available as branded generic drug in a 25-mg tablet. Some pharmacists are unfamiliar with the availability of carbidopa as a single-entity product, and most pharmacies do not typically stock it on their shelves but can obtain it from their distributors in a day or 2.

Summary

There are no clinical trials of 5HTP in youth with depression, but the low cost and over-the-counter availability might make it attractive to some consumers. The data on adults with depression are insufficient and inconclusive, but initial RCTs look promising (OR 4.1, NNT 2.8). 5HTP has been described here in some detail because so little about it appears in the medical literature, even although clinicians familiar with CAM approaches have used 5HTP to treat depression for years. Many of these physicians view this amino acid as a potentially safer intervention than many pharmaceutical agents. Neuropharmacologically, 5HTP is cleaner than the cleanest SSRI, is more selectively serotonergic, and allows for a stronger stimulation of serotonin pathways with a minimal or collateral (adverse) effects, and it has even stronger and cleaner effects when used with carbidopa. Based on the limited data, there have been no reported cases of increased suicidality, behavioral disinhibition, sexual side effects, weight gain, or withdrawal effects.

The absence of adequate systematic clinical data in adults and youth on 5HTP for depression should give clinicians serious pause. However, as an un-patentable amino acid, it has no prospects of making money for pharmaceutical companies, although it may prove pharmacologically superior because of its high selectivity and specificity relative to SSRIs, and its more favorable side effect profile. 5HTP should be receiving a great deal of attention from researchers. With the reputational damage caused by the eosinophilia-myalgia syndrome now seen in historical perspective, 5HTP is ripe and overdue for renewed investigation in adults and youth.

CLINICAL SUMMARY OF CAM APPROACHES TO TREATING MOOD DISORDERS IN YOUTH

Physical exercise, light therapies, hypericum, SAMe, and 5HTP vary widely in the strength of the evidence base supporting their use as potential treatments for MDD in children and adolescents.

Like the medical literature about all novel therapies, the early published clinical trials tend to be few, small in sample size, open-label or weakly blinded, sometimes controlled (placebo or otherwise), lacking in randomization, heterogeneous in sampled populations, diverse in participant characteristics and entry criteria, unconvincing in diagnostic methodology, inadequate in using too few outcomes measures or too many unvalidated measures, unsystematic in assessment of adverse effects, inappropriately analyzed statistically, unimpressive in results, overly generous in data interpretations, overly enthusiastic (or overly skeptical) in conclusions, unrealistically summarized in their abstracts, and suppressed if outcomes are negative (not submitted by investigators or rejected by journals). Preliminary observations, case series, early clinical trials, and even early RCTs often yield uninterpretable results. This review has skipped over many published but fruitless studies.

Yet, despite often unpersuasive evidence, patterns emerge from these early studies that can be useful, and over time researchers and clinicians will pick through the data, bolster the methodology, and find some valuable additions to the treatment armamentarium. The 5 treatments discussed here are strong candidates for such transformation from marginalized status to established treatments of the future.

These CAM treatments, like all others, will be found to have strengths and weaknesses: They may assume a place in the armamentarium, and we will learn of their limitations. CAM treatments, because they seem to come from outside the standards of practice and the standards of concept, are likely to initially have less research and less extensive clinical experience supporting their use than new pharmaceuticals would. They will not have multi-national pharmaceutical companies driving their research. They are less likely to have large randomized double-blind placebo-controlled trials that evaluate their efficacy and safety.

Looking across the available studies on these putative CAM treatments, it is clear that more research is needed regarding their potential as adjunctive therapies and monotherapies, and not only for mild to moderate MDD in adolescents, who have been the subjects of most of the current studies: We also need short-term studies on preadolescents, severe major depression, and bipolar disorder, and we will need studies on relapse prevention, functionality, quality of life, and general medical health. But the current early data provide some initial guidance for our thinking about these CAM approaches.

Physical Exercise

Physical exercise might not be considered a CAM treatment, except that historically it has been viewed as fanciful to believe that voluntary movement or exertion can treat serious physical or mental illness. In psychiatry, even with the considerable research conducted in adults, it remains controversial to what extent physical exercise can be helpful in treating major depression, especially in severe cases. Many clinicians believe that it can be helpful but have not expanded their treatment approach to include routine recommendations for regular physical exercise, partly because of questions about whether it provides more than modest improvement, partly because they have met with failure in attempting to help adults change their lifestyle, and partly because of the belief that depressed patients cannot consistently perform effortful activities.

In children and adolescents, there are numerous studies and 9 RCTs on the relationship of mood and exercise in the general population. The RCTs suggest that aerobic exercise can moderately improve depressed moods in nonclinical samples of youth, with a moderate effect size of 0.66. Other forms of exercise (strengthening, stretching/flexibility training) seem to have similar although mildly weaker effects. Dose dependency seems likely, although excessive exercise can be a sign of psychopathology. Correlational studies suggest that past exercise is not as important as current exercise in determining current mood, and longitudinal studies suggest that exercise has only a weak role in prevention. Few of these inferences are established, and some are tentative. Overall, there seems to be a bidirectional relationship between exercise and mood in the nonclinical population, with a significant but not strong effect.

There is only 1 small RCT on adolescents with MDD, which was encouraging but lacked placebo controls. The estimated effect size was mild (0.35) compared with flexibility training, but stretching itself may have some clinical value in reducing depressed moods, so a preliminary guesstimate of the effect size of physical exercise compared with placebo in youths with MDD might be about 0.3 to 0.6, which is similar to findings regarding exercise effects in adults with MDD. Several placebo-controlled RCTs are needed to establish an effect size in youth with MDD. Given its low side effect burden, the use of physical exercise as an adjunctive therapy for MDD can easily be justified, especially in view of its value for general health, regardless of its effects on mood. Empirical studies are needed to help guide clinicians struggling to figure out how to help youth (and adults) increase their levels of physical exercise. In the meantime, some clinicians may question whether the effect size of physical exercise on depression is large enough to justify the required expenditure of effort by their patients especially for patients with depression. It is promising that the 2 available studies in youth with MDD suggest that they can be sustained in exercise protocols, at least in research settings.

Light Therapies

Two small RCTs of light therapy on MDD also show encouraging effects in adolescents with mild or moderate depression, and the effects were apparent within 1 to 2 weeks. Two additional small RCTs suggest its value in treating delayed sleep-phase disorder, a condition that mimics depression, and in restrictive eating disorder. Youth, especially young children, might find too taxing to sit for 30 to 60 minutes next to a bright light box, but adherence problems with light box therapy might speculatively be fully addressed by the use of dawn simulation.

Hypericum

St. John's wort looks promising in 3 open-label studies, but rigorous data are needed to assess whether the preliminary findings of a reasonably strong and rapid (1-week to 2-week) response are substantive. The adverse effects and drug interactions of hypericum are similar to those seen with pharmaceutical antidepressants, but its use is complicated by the product variability and unpredictability of these herbal extracts. The clinical problems resulting from this lack of product standardization cannot be fully managed by the consistent use of a single brand product, because of proven batch-to-batch variability.

SAMe

SAMe has been documented as an efficacious treatment in adults. The lack of reimbursement by insurance companies for this inexpensive efficacious antidepressant in adults is indefensible. Just as remarkably, there is only 1 small open-label trial on 3 youths, and it too suggests a rapid onset of action of antidepressant effects. Brand selection is critical for this treatment, given its hygroscopicity. SAMe is easy to use, and it needs to be examined in controlled trials in youth with depression (and also for ADHD).

5HTP

Despite being more selectively serotonergic than the most selective SSRI, 5HTP has not been investigated in placebo-controlled RCTs for treating depression in adults or youth. It has been examined in open-label studies in other childhood conditions, including sleep terrors, and in child psychiatric research, in which its hormonal effects have been used as a biological marker of serotonergic activity. The lengthy delay in research that resulted from the now historically remote period of defective product synthesis was appropriate at the time, but it is now long overdue to end. Given its clean neuropharmacologic profile, 5HTP deserves investigation to assess its potential as an antidepressant for adults and youth, as well as for the other numerous indications for SSRIs.

The evidence supporting these treatments is summarized in some accompanying tables: **Table 1** gives a condensed explanation of a system for grading new clinical treatments, developed by United States Preventive Services Task Force (USPSTF). For each treatment, a grade is assigned to the quality of evidence in the medical literature evaluating that treatment, and a second grade is assigned to the strength of clinical recommendations that can be supported by that research. Using the modification of the USPSTF system described in **Table 1**, **Table 2** gives an evidenced-based summary of the 5 CAM interventions for depression in youth discussed here, distinguishing between effects on depressive moods in a community sample of normal youth and the effects on youth with MDD, based on published evidence in the medical literature. **Table 3** displays my own personal opinions of the value of these interventions for treating MDD in youth, based partly on the published evidence base, partly on my clinical experience, and partly on respected colleagues' observations.

There are additional putative CAM treatments for major depression in youth that are covered in other articles of the *Child and Adolescent Psychiatry Clinics of North America*. In a forthcoming issue on CAM, several treatment options from nutritional psychopharmacology are reviewed, including omega-3 fatty acids and micronutrients (vitamins and minerals), including single-nutrient treatments (such as folate and vitamin D) as well as broad-spectrum micronutrient approaches. Other important interventions with potential antidepressant properties are considered, including

Table 1
Explanation of modified USPSTF grading system used in Tables 2 and 3

Tables 2 and 3 use a modified form of the USPSTF system

Each treatment is assigned a grade for quality of evidence and a grade for strength of recommendations

The quality of evidence grade is a qualitative ranking of the strength of the published evidence in the medical literature regarding a treatment:
   Good: consistent benefit in well-conducted studies in different populations
   Fair: data show positive effects, but weak, limited, or indirect evidence
   Poor: cannot show benefit because of data weakness

The strength of recommendations grade provides a qualitative ranking of the clinical recommendations that can be drawn from findings of the studies:
   Insufficient data
   Recommend against (fair evidence of ineffectiveness or harm)
   Neutral (fair evidence for, but seems risky)
   Recommend (fair evidence of benefit and of safety)
   Recommend strongly (good evidence of benefit and safety)

Table 2
Treatment evaluations based on published medical evidence: quality of evidence/strength of recommendations (USPSTF grades)

Treatment	Depressed Moods in Normal Youth		Psychiatric Disorders in Youth		Cost
	USPSTF Grades	Data	USPSTF Grades	Data	
Physical exercise	Fair/ recommend	9 RCTs	Poor/insufficient data	1 RCT without placebo on MDD	Variable
Light therapy	No data		Poor/insufficient data	1 RCT on winter *MDD*	$100–$500 for device
			Poor/insufficient data	1 RCT on nonseasonal MDD	
			Poor/insufficient data	1 RCT on delayed sleep-phase disorder	
			Poor/insufficient data	1 RCT on restrictive eating disorder	
St. John's wort	No data		Poor/insufficient data	2 adequate open-label studies on MDD	$1–$2 daily for 900–1800 mg dose
SAMe	No data		Poor/insufficient data	1 small open-label case series on MDD	$1.50–$3 daily for 800 mg dose
5HTP	No data		No data		$1 daily for 200–400 mg dose ($2.50 if used with carbidopa)

Table 3
Treatment evaluations based on author's personal opinion: quality of evidence/strength of recommendations (USPSTF grades)

Treatment	Depressive Disorders in Youth	Author's Clinical Opinion
Physical exercise	Fair/recommend	Can be useful as adjunctive therapy, although modestly, and can be difficult to institute or maintain
Light therapy	Fair/recommend	Adjunctive therapy for winter MDD, perhaps also for nonseasonal depression; prefer dawn simulator
St. John's wort	No data	Conventional drugs are pharmacologically cleaner and have more predictable effects; numerous drug interactions
SAMe	No data	Can be useful for MDD (also for ADHD), but anxiety may increase (limiting dose increases and effectiveness)
5HTP	No data	Very helpful for MDD, anxiety disorders, obsessive compulsive disorder, insomnia, and carbohydrate craving

EEG biofeedback (ie, alpha asymmetry neurofeedback), mindfulness-based stress reduction, transcendental meditation, progressive muscle relaxation, relaxation therapy, massage, yoga, and music therapy. Acupuncture is not discussed because there is little written about its use for treating depression in youth, even though recent RCTs suggest its value as a monotherapy or as an adjunctive therapy to SSRIs for treating MDD in adults.[155-157] Pet therapy and aromatherapy are also not discussed because of a lack of data regarding youth with MDD, even although these methods might be particularly suitable and acceptable to young children.

All 5 of these putative antidepressant treatments discussed in this article require monitoring for the possible induction of suicide or mania, with the possible exception of exercise. Despite their easy availability to the public and the possible option for self-administration, all of these treatments are best conducted under medical supervision and monitoring. Families may not initially understand that psychiatric disorders in youth require multidimensional interventions, not self-help or self-treatment, even if a component of the treatment is generally available to all.

Again, clinicians who might be tempted to use these treatments, despite the paucity of data in youth, should reserve these treatments for patients or families who cannot reconcile themselves to the use of pharmaceuticals, who strongly prefer nonpharmaceutical treatments, who have failed on multiple conventional antidepressants, or who lack insurance and have limited financial resources to support conventional treatment. Even in such cases, it is sensible practice to ensure that the patient and/or family understand the significance of their decision to use a weakly documented alternative treatment before trying standard-of-practice treatments. It is clinically and legally critical to restrict use of these treatments to those cases in which informed consent is genuine, valid, and carefully documented in the patient's record. Such nonconventional treatments should be used exclusively when the acuity and severity of the clinical situation are mild enough to allow a potential delay in starting conventional treatment.

EMBRACING NEW TECHNIQUES, CONSERVING OLD PRINCIPLES

Unlike many treatments commonly used in psychiatry, these 5 CAM interventions are highly attractive to some patients and consumers. A major part of their appeal is that these treatments can be self-administered, providing the beneficiaries with a sense of self-control and independence. There is strong interest based on cost alone: these treatments can be readily purchased at moderate cost (running shoes, a 1-time purchase of a medical device through the Internet, competing products at health food stores). They do not require office visits to see physicians, insurance copayments, time off from work, or the transportation outlays needed to obtain medical supervision. These treatments are usually well tolerated if common sense and reasonable caution are used. These CAM treatments for depression are especially attractive to youths and parents because their use carries a low very level of stigma.

To professionals, the emergence of over-the-counter or self-administered treatments for major mood disorders may be seen as a grave public health danger. Self-treatment, or treatment of children by their parents, does not fit the standard psychiatric model, for many good reasons. Correct diagnosis is a cornerstone of medicine, and many psychiatric disorders are easy to diagnosis incorrectly. Although parents can safely administer many over-the-counter drugs for a variety of medical ailments, the insight and objectivity required for psychiatric diagnosis and treatment are likely to be compromised by the child's illness and perhaps the parent's psychiatric diagnosis or psychological state. Apart from the technical issues involved (eg, differential diagnosis, assessment of suicide risk, identification of adverse treatment effects, optimization of dosage, anticipation and management of drug interactions), physicians play various critical roles in the treatment of youth with psychiatric conditions (**Box 7**). The do-it-yourself approach to treating major depression or bipolar disorder in youth is not likely, certainly in the average case, to go well. There are potential and unavoidable hazards of self-administered treatments for major mood disorders.

These 5 CAM treatments may also complicate concurrent professionally administered psychiatric treatments, especially if patients and their families are casual or covert about informing the psychiatrist about the use of the CAM treatments. The report of 5 children whose psychiatrists were unaware of their use of hypericum,[95] a

---

Box 7
Do-it-yourself over-the-counter treatment of psychiatric disorders by youth or parents?

Even if psychiatric treatments become readily available and trivially easy, young psychiatric patients and their families still need help with

- Awareness of symptoms or severity
- Assessment of suicide risk
- Identification of medical causes and mimics of psychiatric symptoms
- Diagnosis and management of comorbidity
- Education about illness
- Psychological support
- Psychodevelopmental treatment (eg, psychotherapy)
- Fostering reintegration and social functioning
- Diagnosis and treatment of psychiatric disorders in family members (children's parents, parents' children, siblings)
- Education, support, and management counseling for family

herbal treatment with major drug interactions, serves as a warning. Furthermore, a clinician is unable to interpret the effects of a prescribed antidepressant medication without awareness and proper monitoring of covarying treatments with antidepressant effects.

For these reasons, it is incumbent on child and adolescent psychiatrists to be aware and to keep abreast of the expanding knowledge of commonly used CAM treatments.

Like child and adolescent psychopharmacology 30 years ago, clinicians are faced with difficult choices presented by CAM: The adult data suggest potential clinical usefulness of several treatments, although there are mostly inadequate safety and efficacy data in youth. Based on the psychopharmacology experience, it is likely that some child and adolescent psychiatrists will begin to use these treatments based on judgments made for individual children in specific clinical situations, and that researchers may find themselves again in the position of catching up with the clinicians' use or overuse of underresearched treatments. However, unlike the precedent in child psychopharmacology, which largely pursued medications whose effects in adults had been extensively reviewed by the FDA before their marketing, CAM treatments such as hypericum or 5HTP can be viewed as more exploratory because they have never been subjected to the FDA-mandated evaluations of safety and efficacy.

Others of these CAM treatments might not be viewed as alternative in any sense, such as exercise or light therapy. The 5 treatments discussed in this article do not require any particular change in medical worldview, nor do they represent any true challenge to the traditional medical or physiologic models. Yet they seem novel to many practitioners and researchers in child and adolescent psychiatry: It is time that CAM become viewed as a source of candidate treatments in which research is likely to expand the clinical armamentarium.

Physicians recognize that many members of the public are not particularly doctor friendly, or do not have the funds, or do not have a cultural inclination or a family environment that supports seeking psychiatric help. We all know of people like this, and we certainly know that our patients tell us about family members or friends who are like this. For them, self-treatment with these CAM treatments may be the best that they are likely to get, albeit better if received under medical supervision. For these people, both old (the 54% of adults with depression who use CAM, with or without psychiatric involvement) and young, we owe it as part of our public responsibility to be knowledgeable about these treatments and to deepen the knowledge base through research in these treatments.

REFERENCES

1. Kessler RC, Soukup J, Davis RB, et al. The use of complementary and alternative therapies to treat anxiety and depression in the United States. Am J Psychiatry 2001;158(2):289–94.
2. Kessler RC, Davis RB, Foster DF, et al. Long-term trends in the use of complementary and alternative medical therapies in the United States. Ann Intern Med 2001;135(4):262–8.
3. Elkins G, Rajab MH, Marcus J. Complementary and alternative medicine use by psychiatric inpatients. Psychol Rep 2005;96(1):163–6.
4. Spigelblatt L, Laîné-Ammara G, Pless IB, et al. The use of alternative medicine by children. Pediatrics 1994;94(6 Pt 1):811–4.
5. Sawni-Sikand A, Schubiner H, Thomas RL. Use of complementary/alternative therapies among children in primary care pediatrics. Ambul Pediatr 2002;2(2): 99–103.

6. Sanders H, Davis MF, Duncan B, et al. Use of complementary and alternative medical therapies among children with special health care needs in southern Arizona. Pediatrics 2003;111(3):584–7.
7. Loman DG. The use of complementary and alternative health care practices among children. J Pediatr Health Care 2003;17(2):58–63.
8. Yussman SM, Ryan SA, Auinger P, et al. Visits to complementary and alternative medicine providers by children and adolescents in the United States. Ambul Pediatr 2004;4(5):429–35.
9. Freeman MP, Fava M, Lake J, et al. Complementary and alternative medicine in major depressive disorder: the American Psychiatric Association Task Force report. J Clin Psychiatry 2010;71(6):669–81.
10. Rimer J, Dwan K, Lawlor DA, et al. Exercise for depression. Cochrane Database Syst Rev 2012;(7):CD004366.
11. Sallis JF, Prochaska JJ, Taylor WC. A review of correlates of physical activity of children and adolescents. Med Sci Sports Exerc 2000;32(5):963–75.
12. Brosnahan J, Steffen LM, Lytle L, et al. The relation between physical activity and mental health among Hispanic and non-Hispanic white adolescents. Arch Pediatr Adolesc Med 2004;158(8):818–23.
13. Brunet J, Sabiston CM, Chaiton M, et al. The association between past and current physical activity and depressive symptoms in young adults: a 10-year prospective study. Ann Epidemiol 2013;23(1):25–30.
14. Haarasilta LM, Marttunen MJ, Kaprio JA, et al. Correlates of depression in a representative nationwide sample of adolescents (15-19 years) and young adults (20-24 years). Eur J Public Health 2004;14(3):280–5.
15. Hume C, Timperio A, Veitch J, et al. Physical activity, sedentary behavior, and depressive symptoms among adolescents. J Phys Act Health 2011;8(2):152–6.
16. Johnson CC, Murray DM, Elder JP, et al. Depressive symptoms and physical activity in adolescent girls. Med Sci Sports Exerc 2008;40(5):818–26.
17. Motl RW, Birnbaum AS, Kubik MY, et al. Naturally occurring changes in physical activity are inversely related to depressive symptoms during early adolescence. Psychosom Med 2004;66(3):336–42.
18. Sund AM, Larsson B, Wichstrøm L. Role of physical and sedentary activities in the development of depressive symptoms in early adolescence. Soc Psychiatry Psychiatr Epidemiol 2011;46(5):431–41.
19. Tao FB, Xu ML, Kim SD, et al. Physical activity might not be the protective factor for health risk behaviours and psychopathological symptoms in adolescents. J Paediatr Child Health 2007;43(11):762–7.
20. Stiles-Shields EC, Goldschmidt AB, Boepple L, et al. Driven exercise among treatment-seeking youth with eating disorders. Eat Behav 2011;12(4):328–31.
21. Berczik K, Szabó A, Griffiths MD, et al. Exercise addiction: symptoms, diagnosis, epidemiology, and etiology. Subst Use Misuse 2012;47(4):403–17.
22. Fulkerson JA, Sherwood NE, Perry CL, et al. Depressive symptoms and adolescent eating and health behaviors: a multifaceted view in a population-based sample. Prev Med 2004;38(6):865–75.
23. Jacka FN, Pasco JA, Williams LJ, et al. Lower levels of physical activity in childhood associated with adult depression. J Sci Med Sport 2011;14(3):222–6.
24. Jerstad SJ, Boutelle KN, Ness KK, et al. Prospective reciprocal relations between physical activity and depression in female adolescents. J Consult Clin Psychol 2010;78(2):268–72.
25. Rothon C, Edwards P, Bhui K, et al. Physical activity and depressive symptoms in adolescents: a prospective study. BMC Med 2010;8:32.

26. Sabiston CM, O'Loughlin E, Brunet J, et al. Linking depression symptom trajectories in adolescence to physical activity and team sports participation in young adults. Prev Med 2013;56(2):95–8.
27. Larun L, Nordheim LV, Ekeland E, et al. Exercise in prevention and treatment of anxiety and depression among children and young people. Cochrane Database Syst Rev 2006;(3):CD004691.
28. Beffert JW. Aerobic exercise as treatment of depressive symptoms in early adolescents. Dissertation Abstracts International 1994;54(9-A):1994, 3374, USA.
29. Berger BG, Friedmann E, Eaton M. Comparison of jogging, the relaxation response, and group interaction for stress reduction. J Sport Exerc Psychol 1988;10(4):431–47.
30. Goodrich GL. The effects of aerobic fitness training on hostility and depression in a college population. Dissertation Abstracts International 1984;45(6-B):Dec-B.
31. Hilyer JC, Wilson DG, Dillon C, et al. Physical fitness training and counselling as treatment for youthful offenders. J Couns Psychol 1982;29(3):292–303.
32. Roth DL, Holmes DS. Influence of aerobic exercise training and relaxation training on physical and psychologic health following stressful life events. Psychosom Med 1987;49(4):355–65.
33. Nabkasorn C, Miyai N, Sootmongkol A, et al. Effects of physical exercise on depression, neuroendocrine stress hormones and physiological fitness in adolescent females with depressive symptoms. Eur J Public Health 2006;16(2):179–84.
34. Norris R, Carroll D, Cochrane R. The effects of physical activity and exercise training on psychological stress and well-being in an adolescent population. J Psychosom Res 1992;36(1):55–65.
35. Shomaker LB, Tanofsky-Kraff M, Zocca JM, et al. Depressive symptoms and cardiorespiratory fitness in obese adolescents. J Adolesc Health 2012;50(1): 87–92.
36. Petty KH, Davis CL, Tkacz J, et al. Exercise effects on depressive symptoms and self-worth in overweight children: a randomized controlled trial. J Pediatr Psychol 2009;34(9):929–39.
37. French SA, Story M, Perry CL. Self-esteem and obesity in children and adolescents: a literature review. Obes Res 1995;3(5):479–90.
38. Daley AJ, Copeland RJ, Wright NP, et al. Exercise therapy as a treatment for psychopathologic conditions in obese and morbidly obese adolescents: a randomized, controlled trial. Pediatrics 2006;118(5):2126–34.
39. Toulabi T, Khosh Niyat Nikoo M, Amini F, et al. The influence of a behavior modification interventional program on body mass index in obese adolescents. J Formos Med Assoc 2012;111(3):153–9.
40. Brown SW, Welsh MC, Labbé EE, et al. Aerobic exercise in the psychological treatment of adolescents. Percept Mot Skills 1992;74(2):555–60.
41. Cohen-Kahn DD. The effects of a graded mastery weight-training program on depression and overall functioning in patient adolescents. Dissertation Abstracts International 1995;55(8-B):Feb-B.
42. Kanner KD. High versus low-intensity exercise as part of an inpatient treatment program for childhood and adolescent depression. Dissertation Abstracts International 1991;51(8-B):Feb-B.
43. Dopp RR, Mooney AJ, Armitage R, et al. Exercise for adolescents with depressive disorders: a feasibility study. Depress Res Treat 2012;2012:257472.
44. Hughes CW, Trivedi MH, Cleaver J, et al. DATE: depressed adolescents treated with exercise: study rationale and design for a pilot study. Ment Health Phys Act 2009;2(2):76–85.

45. Hoang QB, Mortazavi M. Pediatric overuse injuries in sports. Adv Pediatr 2012;
    59(1):359–83.
46. Ekeland E, Heian F, Hagen KB, et al. Exercise to improve self-esteem in children
    and young people. Cochrane Database Syst Rev 2004;(1):CD003683.
47. Biddle SJ, Asare M. Physical activity and mental health in children and adoles-
    cents: a review of reviews. Br J Sports Med 2011;45(11):886–95.
48. MacMahon JR, Gross RT. Physical and psychological effects of aerobic exer-
    cise in delinquent adolescent males. Am J Dis Child 1988;142(12):1361–6.
49. Erickson KI, Voss MW, Prakash RS, et al. Exercise training increases size of hippo-
    campus and improves memory. Proc Natl Acad Sci U S A 2011;108(7):3017–22.
50. Tremblay MS, LeBlanc AG, Kho ME, et al. Systematic review of sedentary
    behaviour and health indicators in school-aged children and youth. Int J Behav
    Nutr Phys Act 2011;8:98.
51. Dunn AL, Weintraub P. Exercise in the prevention and treatment of adolescent
    depression: a promising but little researched intervention. Am J Lifestyle Med
    2008;2(6):507–18.
52. Metcalf B, Henley W, Wilkin T. Effectiveness of intervention on physical activity of
    children: systematic review and meta-analysis of controlled trials with objec-
    tively measured outcomes (EarlyBird 54). BMJ 2012;345:e5888.
53. Dobbins M, Husson H, DeCorby K, et al. School-based physical activity
    programs for promoting physical activity and fitness in children and adolescents
    aged 6 to 18. Cochrane Database Syst Rev 2013;2:CD007651.
54. Ortega FB, Ruiz JR, Castillo MJ, et al. Physical fitness in childhood and adoles-
    cence: a powerful marker of health. Int J Obes (Lond) 2008;32(1):1–11.
55. Terman M, Terman JS. Controlled trial of naturalistic dawn simulation and nega-
    tive air ionization for seasonal affective disorder. Am J Psychiatry 2006;163(12):
    2126–33.
56. Golden RN, Gaynes BN, Ekstrom RD, et al. The efficacy of light therapy in the
    treatment of mood disorders: a review and meta-analysis of the evidence. Am
    J Psychiatry 2005;162(4):656–62.
57. Mghir R, Vincent J. Phototherapy of seasonal affective disorder in an adolescent
    female. J Am Acad Child Adolesc Psychiatry 1991;30(3):440–2.
58. Magnusson A. Light therapy to treat winter depression in adolescents in
    Iceland. J Psychiatry Neurosci 1998;23(2):118–22.
59. Sonis WA, Yellin AM, Garfinkel BD, et al. The antidepressant effect of light in
    seasonal affective disorder of childhood and adolescence. Psychopharmacol
    Bull 1987;23(3):360–3.
60. Swedo SE, Allen AJ, Glod CA, et al. A controlled trial of light therapy for the
    treatment of pediatric seasonal affective disorder. J Am Acad Child Adolesc
    Psychiatry 1997;36(6):816–21.
61. Niederhofer H, von Klitzing K. Bright light treatment as mono-therapy of non-
    seasonal depression for 28 adolescents. Int J Psychiatry Clin Pract 2012;
    16(3):233–7.
62. Gradisar M, Dohnt H, Gardner G, et al. A randomized controlled trial of
    cognitive-behavior therapy plus bright light therapy for adolescent delayed
    sleep phase disorder. Sleep 2011;34(12):1671–80.
63. Janas-Kozik M, Krzystanek M, Stachowicz M, et al. Bright light treatment of
    depressive symptoms in patients with restrictive type of anorexia nervosa.
    J Affect Disord 2011;130(3):462–5.
64. Okawa M. Delayed sleep phase syndrome and depression. Sleep Med 2011;
    12(7):621–2.

65. Thorpy MJ, Korman E, Spielman AJ, et al. Delayed sleep phase syndrome in adolescents. J Adolesc Health Care 1988;9(1):22–7.
66. van Geijlswijk IM, Korzilius HP, Smits MG. The use of exogenous melatonin in delayed sleep phase disorder: a meta-analysis. Sleep 2010;33(12):1605–14.
67. Ash JB, Piazza E, Anderson JL. Light therapy in the clinical management of an eating-disordered adolescent with winter exacerbation. Int J Eat Disord 1998; 23(1):93–7.
68. Krysta K, Krzystanek M, Janas-Kozik M, et al. Bright light therapy in the treatment of childhood and adolescence depression, antepartum depression, and eating disorders. J Neural Transm 2012;119(10):1167–72.
69. Schwartz PJ, Brown C, Wehr TA, et al. Winter seasonal affective disorder: a follow-up study of the first 59 patients of the National Institute of Mental Health Seasonal Studies Program. Am J Psychiatry 1996;153(8):1028–36.
70. Schwitzer J, Neudorfer C, Blecha HG, et al. Mania as a side effect of phototherapy. Biol Psychiatry 1990;28:532–4.
71. Kantor DA, Browne M, Ravindran A, et al. Manic-like response to phototherapy. Can J Psychiatry 1991;36(9):697–8.
72. Chan PK, Lam RW, Perry KF. Mania precipitated by light therapy for patients with SAD. J Clin Psychiatry 1994;55(10):454.
73. Meesters Y, van Houwelingen CA. Rapid mood swings after unmonitored light exposure. Am J Psychiatry 1998;155(2):306.
74. Grundmann O, Lv Y, Kelber O, et al. Mechanism of St. John's wort extract (STW3-VI) during chronic restraint stress is mediated by the interrelationship of the immune, oxidative defense, and neuroendocrine system. Neuropharmacology 2010;58(4–5):767–73.
75. Wurglics M, Westerhoff K, Kaunzinger A, et al. Comparison of German St. John's wort products according to hyperforin and total hypericin content. J Am Pharm Assoc (Wash) 2001;41(4):560–6.
76. Linde K, Berner MM, Kriston L. St John's wort for major depression. Cochrane Database Syst Rev 2008;(4):CD000448.
77. Kasper S, Caraci F, Forti B, et al. Efficacy and tolerability of hypericum extract for the treatment of mild to moderate depression. Eur Neuropsychopharmacol 2010;20(11):747–65.
78. Hübner WD, Kirste T. Experience with St John's Wort (*Hypericum perforatum*) in children under 12 years with symptoms of depression and psychovegetative disturbances. Phytother Res 2001;15(4):367–70.
79. Findling RL, McNamara NK, O'Riordan MA, et al. An open-label pilot study of St. John's wort in juvenile depression. J Am Acad Child Adolesc Psychiatry 2003; 42(8):908–14.
80. Simeon J, Nixon MK, Milin R, et al. Open-label pilot study of St. John's wort in adolescent depression. J Child Adolesc Psychopharmacol 2005;15(2):293–301.
81. Fegert JM, Kölch M, Zito JM, et al. Antidepressant use in children and adolescents in Germany. J Child Adolesc Psychopharmacol 2006;16(1–2):197–206.
82. Hoffmann F, Glaeske G, Petermann F, et al. Outpatient treatment in German adolescents with depression: an analysis of nationwide health insurance data. Pharmacoepidemiol Drug Saf 2012;21(9):972–9.
83. Trautmann-Sponsel RD, Dienel A. Safety of Hypericum extract in mildly to moderately depressed outpatients: a review based on data from three randomized, placebo-controlled trials. J Affect Disord 2004;82(2):303–7.
84. Ferko N, Levine MA. Evaluation of the association between St. John's wort and elevated thyroid-stimulating hormone. Pharmacotherapy 2001;21(12):1574–8.

85. Hauben M. The association of St. John's wort with elevated thyroid-stimulating hormone. Pharmacotherapy 2002;22(5):673–5.
86. Haller CA, Meier KH, Olson KR. Seizures reported in association with use of dietary supplements. Clin Toxicol (Phila) 2005;43(1):23–30.
87. Ivetic V, Trivic S, Pogancev MK, et al. Effects of St John's wort (*Hypericum perforatum* L.) extracts on epileptogenesis. Molecules 2011;16(9):8062–75.
88. Etemad L, Heidari MR, Heidari M, et al. Investigation of *Hypericum perforatum* extract on convulsion induced by picrotoxin in mice. Pak J Pharm Sci 2011; 24(2):233–6.
89. Coskun I, Tayfun Uzbay I, Ozturk N, et al. Attenuation of ethanol withdrawal syndrome by extract of *Hypericum perforatum* in Wistar rats. Fundam Clin Pharmacol 2006;20(5):481–8.
90. Hosseinzadeh H, Karimi GR, Rakhshanizadeh M. Anticonvulsant effect of *Hypericum perforatum*: role of nitric oxide. J Ethnopharmacol 2005;98(1–2):207–8.
91. Karalapillai DC, Bellomo R. Convulsions associated with an overdose of St John's wort. Med J Aust 2007;186(4):213–4.
92. Food and Drug Administration MedWatch Safety Alert 2004. Public health advisory: suicidality in children and adolescents being treated with antidepressant medications. Available at: http://www.fda.gov/Drugs/DrugSafety/PostmarketDrug SafetyInformationforPatientsandProviders/DrugSafetyInformationforHeathcare Professionals/PublicHealthAdvisories/ucm161696.htm. Accessed May 10, 2013.
93. Food and Drug Administration News Release. FDA proposes new warnings about suicidal thinking, behavior in young adults who take antidepressant medications. 2007. Available at: http://www.publiccounsel.net/Training/CAFL/ pdf/Medical_Treatment/Clinical/FDA_Update_on_Antidepressant_Use_in_ Children.pdf. Accessed May 10, 2013.
94. Rahimi R, Abdollahi M. An update on the ability of St. John's wort to affect the metabolism of other drugs. Expert Opin Drug Metab Toxicol 2012;8(6):691–708.
95. Walter G, Rey JM. Use of St. John's Wort by adolescents with a psychiatric disorder. J Child Adolesc Psychopharmacol 1999;9(4):307–11.
96. Anderson OS, Sant KE, Dolinoy DC. Nutrition and epigenetics: an interplay of dietary methyl donors, one-carbon metabolism and DNA methylation. J Nutr Biochem 2012;23(8):853–9.
97. Baldessarini RJ. Neuropharmacology of S-adenosyl-L-methionine. Am J Med 1987;83(5A):95–103.
98. Bottiglieri T. Ademetionine (S-adenosylmethionine) neuropharmacology: implications for drug therapies in psychiatric and neurological disorders. Expert Opin Investig Drugs 1997;6(4):417–26.
99. Schaller JL, Thomas J, Bazzan AJ. SAMe use in children and adolescents [letter]. Eur Child Adolesc Psychiatry 2004;13(5):332–4.
100. Chitiva H, Audivert F, Alvarez C. Suicide attempt by self-burning associated with ingestion of S-adenosylmethionine: a review of the literature and case report. J Nerv Ment Dis 2012;200(1):99–101.
101. Shekim WO, Antun F, Hanna GL, et al. S-adenosyl-L-methionine (SAM) in adults with ADHD, RS: preliminary results from an open trial. Psychopharmacol Bull 1990;26(2):249–53.
102. Navon D, Shwed U. The chromosome 22q11.2 deletion: from the unification of biomedical fields to a new kind of genetic condition. Soc Sci Med 2012;75(9): 1633–41.
103. Baker K, Vorstman JA. Is there a core neuropsychiatric phenotype in 22q11.2 deletion syndrome? Curr Opin Neurol 2012;25(2):131–7.

104. Niklasson L, Rasmussen P, Oskarsdóttir S, et al. Autism, ADHD, mental retardation and behavior problems in 100 individuals with 22q11 deletion syndrome. Res Dev Disabil 2009;30(4):763–73.

105. Green T, Weinberger R, Diamond A, et al. The effect of methylphenidate on prefrontal cognitive functioning, inattention, and hyperactivity in velocardiofacial syndrome. J Child Adolesc Psychopharmacol 2011; 21(6):589–95.

106. Green T, Steingart L, Frisch A, et al. The feasibility and safety of S-adenosyl-L-methionine (SAMe) for the treatment of neuropsychiatric symptoms in 22q11.2 deletion syndrome: a double-blind placebo-controlled trial. J Neural Transm 2012;119(11):1417–23.

107. Shaw K, Turner J, Del Mar C. Tryptophan and 5-hydroxytryptophan for depression. Cochrane Database Syst Rev 2001;(3):CD003198.

108. Shaw K, Turner J, Del Mar C. Are tryptophan and 5-hydroxytryptophan effective treatments for depression? A meta-analysis. Aust N Z J Psychiatry 2002;36(4): 488–91.

109. Farinelli S, Mariani A, Grimaldi A, et al. Eosinophilia-myalgia syndrome associated with 5-OH-tryptophan: description of a case. Recenti Prog Med 1991; 82(7–8):381–4 [in Italian].

110. Michelson D, Page SW, Casey R, et al. An eosinophilia-myalgia syndrome related disorder associated with exposure to L-5-hydroxytryptophan. J Rheumatol 1994;21(12):2261–5.

111. Sternberg EM, Van Woert MH, Young SN, et al. Development of a scleroderma-like illness during therapy with L-5-hydroxytryptophan and carbidopa. N Engl J Med 1980;303(14):782–7.

112. Lampert A, Joly P, Thomine E, et al. Scleroderma-like syndrome with bullous morphea during treatment with 5-hydroxytryptophan, carbidopa and flunitrazepam. Ann Dermatol Venereol 1992;119(3):209–11 [in French].

113. Das YT, Bagchi M, Bagchi D, et al. Safety of 5-hydroxy-L-tryptophan. Toxicol Lett 2004;150(1):111–22.

114. Allen JA, Peterson A, Sufit R, et al. Post-epidemic eosinophilia-myalgia syndrome associated with L-tryptophan. Arthritis Rheum 2011;63(11):3633–9.

115. Sternberg EM. Pathogenesis of L-tryptophan eosinophilia myalgia syndrome. Adv Exp Med Biol 1996;398:325–30.

116. Murphy DL, Campbell I, Costa JL. Current status of the indoleamine hypothesis of the affective disorders. In: Psychopharmacology: A Generation of Progress. In: Lipton MA, DiMascio A, Killam RF, editors. New York: Raven Press; 1978.

117. d'Elia G, Hanson L, Raotma H. L-tryptophan and 5-hydroxytryptophan in the treatment of depression. A review. Acta Psychiatr Scand 1978;57(3):239–52.

118. van Praag HM. Management of depression with serotonin precursors. Biol Psychiatry 1981;16(3):291–310.

119. Nolen WA, van de Putte JJ, Dijken WA, et al. Treatment strategy in depression. II. MAO inhibitors in depression resistant to cyclic antidepressants: two controlled crossover studies with tranylcypromine versus L-5-hydroxytryptophan and nomifensine. Acta Psychiatr Scand 1988;78(6):676–83.

120. Zarcone V, Kales A, Scharf M, et al. Repeated oral ingestion of 5-hydroxytryptophan: the effect on behavior and sleep processes in two schizophrenic children. Arch Gen Psychiatry 1973;28(6):843–6.

121. Sverd J, Kupietz SS, Winsberg BG, et al. Effects of L-5-hydroxytryptophan in autistic children. J Autism Child Schizophr 1978;8(2):171–80.

122. Longo G, Rudoi I, Iannuccelli M, et al. Treatment of essential headache in developmental age with L-5-HTP (cross over double-blind study versus placebo). Pediatr Med Chir 1984;6(2):241–5 [in Italian].
123. Santucci M, Cortelli P, Rossi PG, et al. L-5-hydroxytryptophan versus placebo in childhood migraine prophylaxis: a double-blind crossover study. Cephalalgia 1986;6(3):155–7.
124. Horvath GA, Selby K, Poskitt K, et al. Hemiplegic migraine, seizures, progressive spastic paraparesis, mood disorder, and coma in siblings with low systemic serotonin. Cephalalgia 2011;31(15):1580–6.
125. Mizuno TI, Yugari Y. Self mutilation in Lesch-Nyhan syndrome [Letter]. Lancet 1974;1(7860):761.
126. Anderson LT, Herrmann L, Dancis J. The effect of L-5-hydroxytryptophan on self-mutilation in Lesch-Nyhan disease: a negative report. Neuropadiatrie 1976;7(4):439–42.
127. Frith CD, Johnston EC, Joseph MH, et al. Double-blind clinical trial of 5-hydroxytryptophan in a case of Lesch-Nyhan syndrome. J Neurol Neurosurg Psychiatry 1976;39(7):656–62.
128. Anders TF, Cann HM, Ciaranello RD, et al. Further observations on the use of 5-hydroxytryptophan in a child with Lesch-Nyhan syndrome. Neuropadiatrie 1978;9(2):157–66.
129. Castells S, Chakrabarti C, Winsberg BG, et al. Effects of L-5-hydroxytryptophan on monoamine and amino acids turnover in the Lesch-Nyhan syndrome. J Autism Dev Disord 1979;9(1):95–103.
130. De Giorgis G, Miletto R, Iannuccelli M, et al. Headache in association with sleep disorders in children: a psychodiagnostic evaluation and controlled clinical study–L-5-HTP versus placebo. Drugs Exp Clin Res 1987;13(7):425–33.
131. Bruni O, Ferri R, Miano S, et al. L-5-Hydroxytryptophan treatment of sleep terrors in children. Eur J Pediatr 2004;163(7):402–7.
132. Kaufman J, Birmaher B, Perel J, et al. Serotonergic functioning in depressed abused children: clinical and familial correlates. Biol Psychiatry 1998;44(10):973–81.
133. Birmaher B, Kaufman J, Brent DA, et al. Neuroendocrine response to 5-hydroxy-L-tryptophan in prepubertal children at high risk of major depressive disorder. Arch Gen Psychiatry 1997;54(12):1113–9.
134. Campo JV, Dahl RE, Williamson DE, et al. Gastrointestinal distress to serotonergic challenge: a risk marker for emotional disorder? J Am Acad Child Adolesc Psychiatry 2003;42(10):1221–6.
135. Magnussen I, Engbaek F. The effects of aromatic amino acid decarboxylase inhibitors on plasma concentrations of 5-hydroxytryptophan in man. Acta Pharmacol Toxicol (Copenh) 1978;43(1):36–42.
136. Gijsman HJ, van Gerven JM, de Kam ML, et al. Placebo-controlled comparison of three dose-regimens of 5-hydroxytryptophan challenge test in healthy volunteers. J Clin Psychopharmacol 2002;22(2):183–9.
137. Brodie H, Sack R, Siever L. Clinical studies of L-5-hydroxytryptophan in depression. In: Barchas J, Usdin E, editors. Serotonin and behavior. New York: Academic Press; 1973. p. 549–59.
138. Westenberg HG, Gerritsen TW, Meijer BA, et al. Kinetics of I-5-hydroxytryptophan in healthy subjects. Psychiatry Res 1982;7(3):373–85.
139. Zmilacher K, Battegay R, Gastpar M. L-5-hydroxytryptophan alone and in combination with a peripheral decarboxylase inhibitor in the treatment of depression. Neuropsychobiology 1988;20(1):28–35.

140. Matussek N, Angst J, Benkert O, et al. The effect of L-5-hydroxytryptophan alone and in combination with a decarboxylase inhibitor (Ro-4-4602) in depressive patients. Adv Biochem Psychopharmacol 1974;11(0):399–404.

141. Angst J, Woggon B, Schoepf J. The treatment of depression with L-5-hydroxytryptophan versus imipramine. Results of two open and one double-blind study. Arch Psychiatr Nervenkr 1977;224(2):175–86.

142. Mendlewicz J, Youdim MB. Antidepressant potentiation of 5-hydroxytryptophan by L-deprenil in affective illness. J Affect Disord 1980;2(2):137–46.

143. van Praag HM. Studies in the mechanism of action of serotonin precursors in depression. Psychopharmacol Bull 1984;20(3):599–602.

144. Byerley WF, Judd LL, Reimherr FW, et al. 5-Hydroxytryptophan: a review of its antidepressant efficacy and adverse effects. J Clin Psychopharmacol 1987; 7(3):127–37.

145. Hoehn-Saric R, Harris GJ, Pearlson JD, et al. A fluoxetine-induced frontal lobe syndrome in an obsessive-compulsive patient. J Clin Psychiatry 1991;52:131–3.

146. Garland EJ, Baerg EA. Amotivational syndrome associated with selective serotonin reuptake inhibitors in children and adolescents. J Child Adolesc Psychopharmacol 2001;11(2):181–6.

147. Reinblatt SP, Riddle MA. Selective serotonin reuptake inhibitor-induced apathy: a pediatric case series. J Child Adolesc Psychopharmacol 2006;16(1–2): 227–33.

148. Pranzatelli MR, Tate E, Huang Y, et al. Neuropharmacology of progressive myoclonus epilepsy: response to 5-hydroxy-L-tryptophan. Epilepsia 1995;36(8): 783–91.

149. Norcliffe-Kaufmann L, Martinez J, Axelrod F, et al. Hyperdopaminergic crises in familial dysautonomia: A randomized trial of carbidopa. Neurology 2013;80(17): 1611–7.

150. Lopci E, D'Ambrosio D, Nanni C, et al. Feasibility of carbidopa premedication in pediatric patients: a pilot study. Cancer Biother Radiopharm 2012;27(10): 729–33.

151. Müller EE, Locatelli V, Cella S, et al. Prolactin-lowering and -releasing drugs. Mechanisms of action and therapeutic applications. Drugs 1983;25(4):399–432.

152. Meltzer HY, Lowy M, Robertson A, et al. Effect of 5-hydroxytryptophan on serum cortisol levels in major affective disorders. III. Effect of antidepressants and lithium carbonate. Arch Gen Psychiatry 1984;41(4):391–7.

153. Smarius LJ, Jacobs GE, Hoeberechts-Lefrandt DH, et al. Pharmacology of rising oral doses of 5-hydroxytryptophan with carbidopa. J Psychopharmacol 2008; 22(4):426–33.

154. Brod LS, Aldred JL, Nutt JG. Are high doses of carbidopa a concern? A randomized, clinical trial in Parkinson's disease. Mov Disord 2012;27(6):750–3.

155. Andreescu C, Glick RM, Emeremni CA, et al. Acupuncture for the treatment of major depressive disorder: a randomized controlled trial. J Clin Psychiatry 2011;72(8):1129–35.

156. Qu SS, Huang Y, Zhang ZJ, et al. A 6-week randomized controlled trial with 4-week follow-up of acupuncture combined with paroxetine in patients with major depressive disorder. J Psychiatr Res 2013;47(6):726–32.

157. Wu J, Yeung AS, Schnyer R, et al. Acupuncture for depression: a review of clinical applications. Can J Psychiatry 2012;57(7):397–405.

Autism
Biomedical Complementary Treatment Approaches

Robert L. Hendren, DO

KEYWORDS

- Autism • Complementary and alternative treatment • Integrative treatment
- Biomedical treatment

KEY POINTS

- Families commonly seek alternative and complementary biomedical treatments with children with autistic spectrum disorders (ASD).
- Although there are many biomedical CAM treatments in use, there is little evidence from well-conducted randomized controlled trials (RCT) to support claims of efficacy or safety.
- A potential rationale for biomedical CAM treatments in autism is their potential beneficial effect on epigenetic processes, which are increasingly shown to play a role in the gene-environment interactions underlying the development of ASD.
- Three agents with a rationale for use with ASD, at least one RCT showing efficacy, and safety data include melatonin, omega-3, and micronutrients.
- Additional agents with promise include N-acetylcysteine and methylcobalamin (methyl B12), digestive enzymes, and memantine.
- Care providers should be prepared to thoughtfully discuss biomedical CAM treatments with families to help them make informed decisions regarding the best options for their child and for their family's values.

INTRODUCTION

This article provides an overview of the biomedical subgroup of complementary and alternative medicine (CAM) treatments for autism spectrum disorders (ASD). These biomedical treatments include a variety of natural products, such as vitamins and minerals, melatonin, and digestive enzymes; procedures, such as neurofeedback and

Disclosures: Within the past year, the author has received research grants from Forest Pharmaceuticals, Inc; Bristol Meyer Squibb; Otsuka America Pharmaceutical, Inc; Curemark; BioMarin; Autism Speaks; the Vitamin D Council; and NIMH. The author is on an advisory board for BioMarin, Forest, Janssen Pharmaceutical, and the Autism Speaks Treatment Advisory Board. The author is not on any speakers bureaus.
Child and Adolescent Psychiatry, Department of Psychiatry, University of California, San Francisco, 401 Parnassus Avenue, LP-360, San Francisco, CA 94143-0984, USA
E-mail address: Robert.Hendren@ucsf.edu

chelation; some conventional medications that are being examined for new applications in treating autism, such as antifungals and memantine; diets; and nutraceuticals. Nutraceutical agents are foods or food products that purportedly provide health and medical benefits, including the prevention and treatment of disease. Biomedical CAM treatments are integrative in nature, and most of them can be used in combination with conventional treatments for autism.

The author does not review the large number of CAM treatments that are less biomedical in nature, such as mind/body approaches; body-based practices, such as physical manipulation; or alternative medical systems, such as Ayurvedic or traditional Chinese medicine, despite the promising suggestive findings for some of these treatments.

This article begins with a description of the evolving understanding of the cause of ASD and how the recent shift in the etiologic paradigm is leading to increasing assessment of treatment targets and the use of biomedical and CAM treatments. Many of the potential biomedical CAM treatments are listed, and the ones with the most evidence or most focus of public interest are reviewed briefly, along with a discussion of the research models necessary to identify which children will be most likely to respond to which treatments. Finally, a model is discussed for working with families who have a member with an ASD when considering biomedical/CAM treatments. When the term *autism* is used alone, it refers to *autistic disorder* as defined in the *Diagnostic and Statistical Manual of Mental Disorders* (Fourth Edition). When *ASD* is used, it refers to the spectrum of autism disorders from mild to severe.

Complementary and alternative treatments are commonly used. Although 12% of children and adolescents in the United States use CAM treatments,[1] up to 70% of children with ASD are reported to use some form of biologic treatment (either CAM or conventional),[2] and an even higher percentage (up to 74%) of children with recently diagnosed autism use only CAM and not conventional psychopharmacologic agents.[3] The main reasons for families' choice of CAM were related to concerns with the safety and side effects of prescribed medications.[3] Families are reported to expect their primary care physicians to have knowledge about CAM treatments,[4] yet many physicians do not feel knowledgeable about them.

Cause of Autism and the Biomedical Concept

The cause of autism is widely accepted to be strongly genetic in origin, but the increasing prevalence and recent studies of the genetics of autism[5,6] suggest that the cause of autism is also related to gene-by-environment interactions expressed through or manifest in epigenetic processes. Epigenetics refers to the reversible regulation of various genomic functions, independent of DNA sequence, mediated principally through DNA methylation, chromatin sequence, and RNA-mediated gene expression.[7] The related endophenotypes (measurable components along the epigenetic pathway between the genotype and the distal symptom, personal characteristic, or phenotype) are simple biologic aspects of a disease that can be observed in unaffected relatives with a similar endophenotype at a higher rate than in the general population[8] and that are potentially reversible through nutrition, social factors, behavioral interventions, and drugs.[9] Executive and frontal lobe functions shared by family members may be examples.

In autism, this process of gene-environment interaction and the resulting endophenotypes might be viewed schematically as a model in which the layers of the earth represent the expression of the genotype into various types of the phenotype (**Fig. 1**). The surface of the earth represents the personal expression and symptoms we see (phenotype), and the core of the earth represents the genes of that person

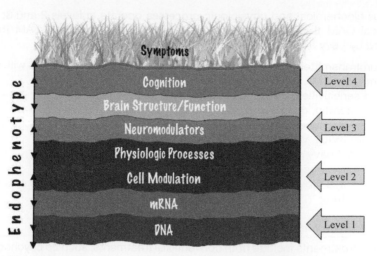

Fig. 1. Surface (phenotype) to core (genotype) model of endophenotype.

(genotype). In between is the complex and interactive layering of developmental processes that represent the endophenotype. Interventions targeting the surface level 4 might include behavioral interventions, such as applied behavior analysis and the external provision of structure. Levels 3 to 4 can be targeted with occupational therapy, physical therapy, speech and language therapy, and cognitive behavioral therapy; levels 3 to 2 with pharmacotherapy; deeper into levels 3 and 2 with biomedical and CAM therapies; and level 1 with treatments that result in gene modification.

This middle earth of levels 2 and 3 is the target of biomedical therapy in autism and other neurodevelopmental disorders and entails various active biochemical or physiologic processes such as the following:

- Immune abnormalities/inflammation[10]
- Oxidative stress[11]
- Disturbed methylation[11]
- Mitochondrial dysfunction[12]
- Free fatty acid metabolism[13]
- Excitatory/inhibitory imbalance[14]
- Hormonal effects[15]

Such abnormal epigenetic processes are not found in all people with ASD or may be active only during particular periods of time (**Fig. 2**). Therefore, treatment research should recruit subjects for trials based on the state of their previously validated endophenotypic biomarkers[16] to know if an intervention is targeting an active biomedical process in the subject at that time. For instance, identifying an inflammatory process through a biomarker such as a cytokine abnormality could be entry criteria to a study of an antiinflammatory agent for the treatment of autism. Other biomarkers of the active epigenetic process might be such measures as glutathione (GSH) metabolites, glutamate and γ-aminobutyric acid, magnetic resonance imaging, genomic arrays, and others based on the current gene-by-environment interaction altering the epigenetic process[17] and are discussed further in studies presented later in this article.

Various biochemical and physiologic processes operate at levels 2 and 3; various biomedical CAM therapies can target these processes, including CAM therapies described by Levy and Hyman[18–20]:

- Neurotransmitter production or release (dimethylglycine, vitamin B6 with magnesium, vitamin C, omega-3 fatty acids, St. John's wort)
- Food sensitivities and gastrointestinal function (gluten-free casein-free [GFCF] diets, secretin, digestive enzymes, famotidine [Pepcid], antibiotics)
- Putative immune mechanism or modulators (antifungals, intravenous immunoglobulin [IVIG], vitamin A/cod liver oil)
- Potential heavy metal toxin removal (chelation)
- Methylation (methylcobalamin, folinic acid)
- Nonbiologic (craniosacral manipulation, transcranial magnetic stimulation, acupuncture)

Biomedical Treatments

Biomedical treatments include both conventional treatments, such as psychopharmacological agents, and less studied and less medically accepted treatments, such as nutraceuticals, as well as other types of treatments, including devices like transcranial magnetic stimulation.

Risperidone and aripiprazole are the only medications that the Food and Drug Administration (FDA) has given approval for marketing for the indication of *irritability*

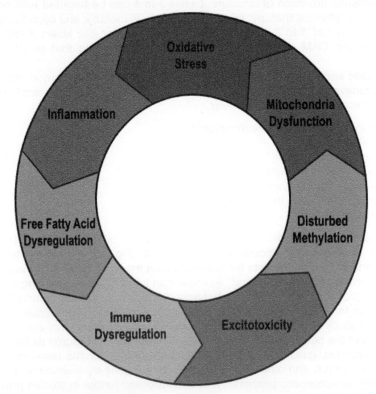

Fig. 2. Endophenotype stress cycle.

associated with autism. Irritability is not a core symptom of autism, and no drug has the FDA's marketing approval for the indication of autism itself or for any core symptom of autism.

Conventional pharmacologic treatments for symptoms associated with ASD include stimulants, antidepressants, antipsychotics, anticonvulsants, and anxiolytics. Each of these agents has been examined for autism-related symptoms in published studies, and comprehensive critical reviews of this literature are available in 2 excellent recent articles.[21,22]

Pharmacologic agents that are not traditionally considered as treatments of ASD or associated symptoms but that have one or more published studies for the treatment of symptoms associated with autism include propranolol,[23] amantadine,[24] D-cyclo-serine,[25] cholinesterase inhibitors,[26] nicotinic agonist,[27] memantine,[28] naltrexone,[29] and buspirone.[30]

The list of potential biomedical CAM treatments is long and most have inadequate evidence to judge potential efficacy. See **Box 1** for a list of most of the biomedical CAM treatments of ASD. Two comprehensive reviews of those treatments with reasonable efficacy data have been recently published.[31,32]

For this short article, the biomedical CAM treatments that have the most published evidence, that have generated the greatest interest or controversy, and/or that nonetheless have significant promise for treating autism or autism-associated symptoms are briefly discussed. These treatments include melatonin, omega-3, injectable methylcobalamin (methyl B12), N-acetylcysteine (NAC), memantine, pancreatic digestive enzymes, micronutrients, immune therapies, and chelation.

Melatonin

Melatonin is an endogenous neurohormone released by the pineal gland in response to decreasing levels of light. It causes drowsiness and sets the body's sleep clock. ASD is associated with a high frequency of sleep problems, and melatonin is increasingly used to help children with ASD fall asleep.[33,34] Rossignol and Frye[35] published a review and meta-analysis of 35 studies. They described reports of abnormalities in melatonin levels in patients with ASD (9 studies: 7 low, 2 high, 4 circadian); significant correlations between melatonin levels and ASD symptoms (4 studies); and gene abnormalities associated with decreased melatonin production (5 studies). Of 18 treatment studies of melatonin, there were 5 randomized controlled trials (RCTs) involving a total of 61 patients treated with nightly doses of 2 to 10 mg. These RCTs showed positive effects on sleep in that sleep duration was increased (44 minutes, Effect Size [ES] = 0.93) and sleep onset latency was decreased (39 minutes, ES = 1.28), but nighttime awakenings were unchanged. The duration of the studies varied between 4 weeks and 4 years. One study suggested a loss of benefit at 4 weeks, whereas the study of 4 years reported continued benefits. The side effects were minimal to none.

Melatonin is one of the best-studied biomedical CAM treatments of ASD. Although small sample sizes, variability in sleep assessments, and lack of follow-up limit the value of these studies in supporting its use, treatment with melatonin has a clear physiologic rationale; and it is sensible, easy, cheap, and safe.

Omega-3 Fatty Acids

Omega-3 long-chain fatty acid supplementation is reasonable to consider because omega-3 fatty acids are essential to brain function and development.[36] They are a critical component of neuronal membranes, they are essential for their optimal functioning, and they serve as substrates for the production of the eicosanoids, such as prostaglandins, which are necessary for cell communication and immune regulation.

Box 1
Potential biomedical CAM treatments of ASD

Pioglitazone hydrochloride (Actos)	Immune therapies
Acupuncture	IVIG
Animal-assisted therapy	L-carnosine
Antibiotics	Magnesium
Antifungals (fluconazole [Diflucan], nystatin)	Melatonin
Antiviral (valacyclovir hydrochloride [Valtrex])	Methylcobalamin (methyl B12)
Amino acids	N-acetylcysteine
Auditory integration therapy (music therapy)	Naltrexone
Chelation	Neurofeedback
Chiropractic	Oxalate (low) diet
Cholestyramine	Oxytocin
Coenzyme Q10	Pyridoxal phosphate
Craniosacral therapy	Probiotics
Curcumin	Ribose and dehydroepiandrosterone
Cyproheptadine	S-adenosyl-methionine
Dehydroepiandrosterone	Secretin
Digestive enzymes	Sensory integration therapy
Dimethylglycine, trimethylglycine	Specific carbohydrate diet
Fatty acids (omega-3)	St. John's wort
5-hydroxytryptophan	Steroids
Folic/folinic acid	Transfer factor
GSH	Vitamin A
GFCF diet	Vitamin B3
Food-allergy treatment	Vitamin B6 with magnesium
Hyperbaric oxygen treatment	Vitamin C
Iron	Zinc
Infliximab (Remicade)	

The two omega-3 fatty acids of primary interest are eicosapentaenoic acid (EPA) and docosahexaenoic acid (DHA). Based on data from other disorders, they might be expected to improve mood, attention, and activity level as well as, conceivably, actual symptoms of autism. Low levels of omega-3 fatty acids have been reported in children with ASD.[37–39]

There have been 4 open trials[35,38,40] and 2 double-blind, placebo-controlled, randomized pilot trials in children with ASD.[41,42] Amminger and colleagues[42] randomized 13 children (aged 5–17 years) to EPA 840 mg and DHA 700 mg daily (n = 7) or placebo (n = 6) for 6 weeks. There were no significant differences between groups on the Aberrant Behavior Checklist, possibly because of the small sample and insufficient power; but omega-3 seemed nominally superior to placebo for stereotypy (Cohen's d = 0.72), hyperactivity (d = 0.71), and inappropriate speech (d = 0.39). In a study by Bent and colleagues,[43] 27 children (aged 3–8 years) with ASD were randomly assigned to 12 weeks of omega-3 fatty acids (1.3 g/d) or an identical placebo. Hyperactivity seemed to improve more in the omega-3 group than in the placebo group, although not with statistical significance (2.7 ± 4.8 vs 0.3 ± 7.2, P = .40). Correlations were found between decreases in the levels of 5 different fatty acids and decreases in hyperactivity, with milder changes in other behaviors. There were no differences in side effects. A larger Internet-based study of omega-3 fatty acid supplementation is currently underway.

With only 2 small placebo-controlled RCTs totaling 38 children, and all 4 open studies without statistically significant effects (possibly a power issue), the evidence is small for omega-3 supplementation in ASD. This effect of omega-3 supplementation on hyperactive behavior might mirror recent suggestions of a modest,[44] though debatable,[45] effect of omega-3 fatty acids in treating attention-deficit hyperactivity disorder (ADHD). Despite the weak evidence and the modest effect, it has a rationale for its use; and it is sensible, easy, inexpensive, and safe.

Methylcobalamin (Methyl B12)

Methyl B12 is a vital cofactor for the regeneration of methionine from homocysteine, by providing methyl groups for metabolic pathways involving transmethylation and transsulfuration. Reduced activity in the transsulfuration pathway can lead to reduced levels of cysteine and GSH, which are crucial antioxidants responsible for minimizing macromolecular damage produced by oxidative stress.

James and colleagues[11] showed that many children with ASD exhibit low levels of GSH and a decreased GSH/GSSG redox ratio. In an open-label trial in 40 children with autism, administration of methyl B12 for 1 month resulted in a significant increase in plasma GSH concentrations, although behavioral assessments were not done in this study.[11] Improvements were noted in social relatedness, language, and behavior problems.

In a recent study, 30 patients completed a 12-week, double-blind RCT of subcutaneously injected methyl B12 at a dosage of 64.5 mcg/kg every 3 days; 22 patients completed the 6-month extension study.[46] The supplement was well tolerated. No statistically significant differences in behavior tests or in GSH status were identified between active and placebo groups. However, 9 (30%) patients demonstrated clinically significant improvement on the Clinical Global Impression–Improvement Scale and at least 2 behavioral and language measures. Improvements in social interaction and language were most consistently reported. Notably, this subgroup of responders exhibited significantly increased concentrations of GSH and GSH/GSSG compared with the nonresponders. This study is the only published RCT, but a new RCT from the same group will be completed in early 2013. Additional research is needed to delineate a subgroup of responders and ascertain a biomarker of response to methyl B12.

Methyl B12 is typically administered at dosages of 64.5 to 75.0 mcg/kg with subcutaneous injections every 2 to 3 days. There are no studies in ASD of oral or nasal methyl B12, which do not maintain consistently high levels and are thought to be less effective. Subcutaneous injectable methyl B12 does seem to be safe. Although initial studies are promising for a subgroup of children with ASD, and subcutaneous injectable methyl B12 supplementation seems to be safe and well tolerated, additional study is needed to determine whether this will become a recommended treatment of ASD. However, despite reasonable cost, with repeated frequent injections, this treatment is not easy to use.

NAC

NAC is a glutamatergic modulator and an antioxidant. There is one published report of a 12-week, double-blind, randomized, placebo-controlled study of NAC in children with autism.[47] Patients (31 boys, 2 girls; aged 3–10 years) were randomized, and NAC was initiated at 900 mg daily for 4 weeks, then 900 mg twice daily for 4 weeks, and 900 mg 3 times daily for 4 weeks. Compared with placebo, oral NAC resulted in significant improvements on the Aberrant Behavior Checklist (ABC) irritability subscale ($P<.001$; d = 0.96) and induced limited side effects. The results are promising, especially because the supplement is well tolerated; but this study will need to be replicated before recommendations can be offered.

Memantine

There are biochemical studies suggesting that aberrant functioning of the N-methyl D-aspartic acid (NMDA) receptor and/or altered glutamate metabolism may play a role in autism. Memantine is a moderate-affinity antagonist of the NMDA glutamate receptor and is hypothesized to potentially modulate learning by blocking excessive glutamate effects that can include neuroinflammatory activity. Its capacity to block glutamate neurotoxicity and neuroinflammatory activity and to stimulate synapse formation makes it an interesting candidate for treating autism. An open-label case series reported significant improvement in language and socialization in children with autism.[28] Memantine is well tolerated in children, and a multisite RCT is currently underway. This treatment could be considered off-label use of a conventional medication approved for the treatment of Alzheimer disorder rather than as a CAM treatment.

Pancreatic Digestive Enzymes

Enzyme deficiencies in children with autism result in a reduced ability to digest protein, which affects the availability of amino acids essential for brain function. There is increasing evidence for a gut-brain connection associated with ASD, at least in some cases.[48] This finding suggests a possible benefit from a comprehensive digestive enzyme supplement with meals to aid digestion of all proteins and peptides, especially for those children with ASD who have gastrointestinal disturbance.

Probiotics (consisting of microorganisms thought to improve digestive health by repopulating the gastrointestinal tract with favorable flora) have also been proposed to improve digestion and gut-brain activity in children with ASD. Some proponents suggest these agents may also help remove toxins and improve immune function.

A double-blind placebo-controlled trial of digestive enzyme supplementation using a 6-month crossover design in 43 children with ASD (aged 3–8 years) did not show any clinically significant improvement of ASD symptoms.[49] A possible effect on improvement in the variety of foods eaten was suggested in the results. A commercially developed product (CM-AT by Curemark) has been specifically developed to target enzyme deficiencies that affect the availability of amino acids in children with autism; fecal chymotrypsin is used as a biomarker. Curemark (www.curemark.com) notes that it has reached its targeted enrollment for a phase III study of a total 170 children with autism at 18 sites. The unpublished Curemark study is interesting, and the FDA is reviewing its findings; but further conclusions await the published results. There are no reported trials of probiotics for ASD.

Micronutrients (Vitamins and Minerals)

Although multivitamin and mineral levels generally are not found to be abnormal in children with autism, biomarkers of general nutritional status have been reported to be associated with autism severity.[50] One open-label study of 44 individuals with autism, aged 2 to 28 years, who were selected because they (or their parents) preferred a natural treatment, reported a benefit.[51] There are only 2 RCT clinical trials of multivitamin/multimineral supplements for children with autism, both from the same group. The first randomized 20 children (aged 3–8 years) and reported the micronutrient supplement yielded significantly better sleep and gastrointestinal symptoms than placebo.[52] Another RCT of an oral vitamin/mineral supplement for 3 months with 141 children and adults with ASD showed an improved nutritional and metabolic status of children with autism, including improvements in methylation, GSH, oxidative stress, sulfation, ATP, NADH, and NADPH.[53] The micronutrient-treated group also had significantly greater improvements on measures of global change ($P = .008$), hyperactivity ($P = .003$), and tantrums ($P = .009$).[53]

Despite limited evidence for the efficacy of vitamin and mineral supplements for autism, there is widespread usage. The promising results from 2 RCTs suggest benefit from a safe, easy to use, and relatively inexpensive agent.

Immune Therapies

Evidence is accumulating that there are subgroups of patients with ASD that have immune deficiencies and signs of autoimmunity, such as atopy.[10] Various approaches have been tried to boost immune function or block autoimmunity. One of the most obvious candidates has been IVIG treatment, and there are now 6 published open-label trials of IVIG treatment with ASD.

In one open-label study, IVIG treatment improved eye contact, speech, behavior, echolalia, and other autistic features.[53] Others have claimed that IVIG treatment led to improvements in gastrointestinal signs and symptoms as well as behavior. Subsequent studies have shown questionable benefits and mixed results for language and behavior.

IVIG is a biomedical treatment whose overall results have been weak, and it carries some significant risks. Other immune-boosting therapies may be of benefit but have not been adequately studied. For future studies, it is unclear if an underlying immunologic dysfunction is present in all individuals with ASD or if treatment trials should target the patients with demonstrable inflammatory changes.

Chelation

Chelation, a process for removing heavy metals from the blood, has been used in treating ASD based on the unproven theory that ASD is caused by heavy metal toxicity; there is no convincing evidence of heavy metal toxicity from biochemical studies in ASD. The hypothesized accumulation of heavy metals, particularly mercury, would presumably be caused by the body's inability to clear the heavy metals, by increased exposure, or both.

Detoxification involves several intermittent courses of oral 2, 3-dimercaptosuccinic acid (DMSA) or the intravenous chelator ethylenediaminetetraacetic acid, with periodic elemental analysis of urine. According to proponents, successful detoxification treatment requires clearing the gastrointestinal tract of harmful dysbiotic flora and bolstering metabolism with essential nutrients, so that the individual can tolerate detoxification.

Two related studies have been published[54,55] involving 65 children with ASD who received one course of DMSA for 3 days. Selected for high urinary excretion of toxic metals following the DMSA administration, 49 were randomly assigned in a double-blind design to receive either 6 additional rounds of DMSA or placebo. DMSA was reportedly well tolerated and resulted in high excretion of heavy metals, normalization of red blood cell GSH, and possibly improved ASD symptoms. Further studies are needed to confirm these results.

Chelation is controversial because of its risks and because of its questionable clinical findings, and the Institute of Medicine recently issued warnings. The most common side effects are diarrhea and fatigue. Less common side effects include abnormal complete blood count, liver function tests, and mineral levels. Renal and hepatic toxicity is possible with oral agents, and seizures have been reported. Some patients may experience a sulfur smell, regression, gastrointestinal symptoms, or rash.

Summary of Biomedical Treatments for Autism and Future Directions

Research on CAM biomedical treatments for autism remains in its early stages, but emerging data suggest several possible directions for current treatments (**Tables 1** and **2**) and future development. Melatonin for sleep induction is supported by 3 of 5 RCTs in children with ASD. Omega-3 fatty acids have 2 positive trending RCTs suggesting the possibility of clinical value for treating hyperactivity associated with ASD, but this might mirror recent findings of the putative efficacy of omega-3 fatty acids in treating ADHD. Methylcobalamin may induce behavioral improvements, according to a single RCT, but the treatment involves repeated injections several times weekly. NAC has one RCT suggesting improvement in irritability. Memantine, which is an established prescription drug treatment for Alzheimer disease, showed encouraging results on language and socialization in one open-label series. Digestive enzyme supplementation is weakly supported by weak data, but a recent unpublished study suggests possible benefit. Micronutrients (multivitamin and multimineral mixtures), based on 2 RCTs, may improve tantrums, hyperactivity, sleep, and gastrointestinal symptoms. IVIGs have mixed findings in open-label trials (no controlled trials), entail medical risks, and require repeated injections. Chelation showed trends toward improvements in sociability, language, and cognition in a single RCT; but again medical risks are significant.

Table 1
Evaluations of biomedical CAM treatments for ASD: the evidence base

Treatment	Quality of Evidence	Strength of Recommendations Based on Data	Evidence Base in Youth
Melatonin	Good	Recommend strongly	18 trials, 5 RCT
Omega-3 fatty acids	Good	Recommend	4 open trials, 2 RCT
Multivitamin/ micronutrients	Fair	Recommend	2 RCTs
NAC	Fair	Neutral/recommend	1 RCT with group significance
Memantine	Fair	Neutral/recommend	3 open trials, ongoing multisite
Digestive enzymes	Poor	Neutral	Anecdotal evidence
Methylcobalamin (methyl B12)	Fair	Neutral	1 RCT w/o significance
Immune therapies intravenous	Poor	Insufficient data	None
Immunoglobulins	Poor	Insufficient data	None
Chelation	Poor	Insufficient data	None

Abbreviation: w/o, without.

Table 2 Evaluation of biomedical CAM treatments for ASD: authors' personal clinical opinion		
Treatment	Strength of Recommendations Based on Published Data	Author's Clinical Recommendations
Melatonin	Reasonably good studies	Very useful
Omega-3 fatty acids	Improvement trends	Suggest always
Multivitamin/micronutrients	Possible benefit	Routinely recommend
NAC	Promising	Suggest
Memantine	Good open label	Frequently consider
Methylcobalamin (methyl B12)	Promising for subgroup	Suggest cautiously
Digestive enzymes	Not good evidence, yet	Suggest for GI symptoms
Immune therapies	No good data	Discourage
IVIG	No good evidence	Discourage
Chelation	Not good evidence	Discourage

Abbreviation: GI, gastrointestinal.

Taken together, none of these treatments are ready for general usage; but some families might elect to try such treatments. It is desirable for practitioners and families to work together to review, evaluate, and perhaps select the treatments that offer the most promise, have a rationale for use, fit with the families' values, and have evidence for safety and possible efficacy.

Multiple levels for intervention in the treatment of ASD are possible. Reviewing and monitoring the levels for intervention assures an integrated approach to autism treatment. A thorough medical assessment includes a review of symptoms, including a possible genetic, neurologic, and gastrointestinal workup and consideration of other medical symptoms when indicated. Applied behavioral analysis approaches, speech and language assessment followed by therapies indicated by these evaluations, and possible occupational therapy should be considered. Education, help in identifying appropriate resources, and overall support is an essential part of the collaborative relationship between the practitioner and the family.

Conventional psychopharmacology should be considered for severe symptoms associated with autism, such as aggression, irritability, and anxiety. Integrated into these interventions should be a thoughtful review and possible use of biomedical CAM treatments, including melatonin for sleep, micronutrients, and omega-3 fatty acids. Other interventions with promise and some safety data include NAC, digestive enzymes, and methylcobalamin.

REFERENCES

1. Birdee GS, Phillips RS, Davis RB, et al. Factors associated with pediatric use of complementary and alternative medicine. Pediatrics 2010;125(2):249–56.
2. Wong HH, Smith RG. Patterns of complementary and alternative medical therapy use in children diagnosed with autism spectrum disorders. J Autism Dev Disord 2006;36(7):901–9.
3. Hanson E, Kalish LA, Bunce E, et al. Use of complementary and alternative medicine among children diagnosed with autism spectrum disorder. J Autism Dev Disord 2007;37(4):628–36.

4. Ben-Arye E, Frenkel M, Klein A, et al. Attitudes toward integration of complementary and alternative medicine in primary care: perspectives of patients, physicians and complementary practitioners. Patient Educ Couns 2008;70(3):395–402.

5. Hallmayer J, Cleveland S, Torres A, et al. Genetic heritability and shared environmental factors among twin pairs with autism. Arch Gen Psychiatry 2011;68(11): 1095–102.

6. Sanders SJ, Murtha MT, Gupta AR, et al. De novo mutations revealed by whole-exome sequencing are strongly associated with autism. Nature 2012;485(7397): 237–41.

7. Jaenisch R, Bird A. Epigenetic regulation of gene expression: how the genome integrates intrinsic and environmental signals. Nat Genet 2003;33(Suppl):245–54.

8. Saresella M, Marventano I, Guerini FR, et al. An autistic endophenotype results in complex immune dysfunction in healthy siblings of autistic children. Biol Psychiatry 2009;66(10):978–84.

9. Rutten BP, Mill J. Epigenetic mediation of environmental influences in major psychotic disorders. Schizophr Bull 2009;35(6):1045–56.

10. Goines P, Van de Water J. The immune system's role in the biology of autism. Curr Opin Neurol 2010;23(2):111–7.

11. James SJ, Melnyk S, Fuchs G, et al. Efficacy of methylcobalamin and folinic acid treatment on glutathione redox status in children with autism. Am J Clin Nutr 2009;89(1):425–30.

12. Frye RE, Rossignol DA. Mitochondrial dysfunction can connect the diverse medical symptoms associated with autism spectrum disorders. Pediatr Res 2011; 69(5 Pt 2):41R–7R.

13. Bell JG, Miller D, MacDonald DJ, et al. The fatty acid compositions of erythrocyte and plasma polar lipids in children with autism, developmental delay or typically developing controls and the effect of fish oil intake. Br J Nutr 2010; 103(8):1160–7.

14. Rubenstein JL. Three hypotheses for developmental defects that may underlie some forms of autism spectrum disorder. Curr Opin Neurol 2010;23(2):118–23.

15. Harony H, Wagner S. The contribution of oxytocin and vasopressin to mammalian social behavior: potential role in autism spectrum disorder. Neurosignals 2010;18(2):82–97.

16. Bent S, Hendren RL. Improving the prediction of response to therapy in autism. Neurotherapeutics 2010;7(3):232–40.

17. Hendren RL, Bertoglio K, Ashwood P, et al. Mechanistic biomarkers for autism treatment. Med Hypotheses 2009;73(6):950–4.

18. Levy SE, Hyman SL. Novel treatments for autistic spectrum disorders. Ment Retard Dev Disabil Res Rev 2005;11(2):131–42.

19. Hyman SL, Levy SE. Introduction: novel therapies in developmental disabilities–hope, reason, and evidence. Ment Retard Dev Disabil Res Rev 2005;11(2): 107–9.

20. Levy SE, Hyman SL. Complementary and alternative medicine treatments for children with autism spectrum disorders. Child Adolesc Psychiatr Clin N Am 2008; 17(4):803–20, ix.

21. Hoffmann TJ, Kvale MN, Hesselson SE, et al. Next generation genome-wide association tool: design and coverage of a high-throughput European-optimized SNP array. Genomics 2011;98(2):79–89 PMID:21565264 PMCID: PMC23146553.

22. McPheeters ML, Warren Z, Sathe N, et al. A systematic review of medical treatments for children with autism spectrum disorders. Pediatrics 2011;127(5): e1312–21.

23. Narayanan A, White CA, Saklayen S, et al. Effect of propranolol on functional connectivity in autism spectrum disorder–a pilot study. Brain Imaging Behav 2010;4(2):189–97.
24. King BH, Wright DM, Handen BL, et al. Double-blind, placebo-controlled study of amantadine hydrochloride in the treatment of children with autistic disorder. J Am Acad Child Adolesc Psychiatry 2001;40(6):658–65.
25. Posey DJ, Kem DL, Swiezy NB, et al. A pilot study of D-cycloserine in subjects with autistic disorder. Am J Psychiatry 2004;161(11):2115–7.
26. Chez MG, Aimonovitch M, Buchanan T, et al. Treating autistic spectrum disorders in children: utility of the cholinesterase inhibitor rivastigmine tartrate. J Child Neurol 2004;19(3):165–9.
27. Deutsch SI, Urbano MR, Neumann SA, et al. Cholinergic abnormalities in autism: is there a rationale for selective nicotinic agonist interventions? Clin Neuropharmacol 2010;33(3):114–20.
28. Chez MG, Burton Q, Dowling T, et al. Memantine as adjunctive therapy in children diagnosed with autistic spectrum disorders: an observation of initial clinical response and maintenance tolerability. J Child Neurol 2007;22(5):574–9.
29. Brown N, Panksepp J. Low-dose naltrexone for disease prevention and quality of life. Med Hypotheses 2009;72(3):333–7.
30. Doyle CA, McDougle CJ. Pharmacotherapy to control behavioral symptoms in children with autism. Expert Opin Pharmacother 2012;13(11):1615–29.
31. Lofthouse N, Hendren R, Hurt E, et al. A review of complementary and alternative treatments for autism spectrum disorders. Autism Res Treat 2012;2012: 870391. http://dx.doi.org/10.1155/2012/870391.
32. Rossignol DA. Novel and emerging treatments for autism spectrum disorders: a systematic review. Ann Clin Psychiatry 2009;21(4):213–36.
33. Miano S, Ferri R. Epidemiology and management of insomnia in children with autistic spectrum disorders. Paediatr Drugs 2010;12(2):75–84.
34. Wirojanan J, Jacquemont S, Diaz R, et al. The efficacy of melatonin for sleep problems in children with autism, fragile X syndrome, or autism and fragile X syndrome. J Clin Sleep Med 2009;5(2):145–50.
35. Rossignol DA, Frye RE. Melatonin in autism spectrum disorders: a systematic review and meta-analysis. Dev Med Child Neurol 2011;53(9):783–92.
36. Freeman MP, Hibbeln JR, Wisner KL, et al. Omega-3 fatty acids: evidence basis for treatment and future research in psychiatry. J Clin Psychiatry 2006;67(12): 1954–67.
37. Bell JG, MacKinlay EE, Dick JR, et al. Essential fatty acids and phospholipase A2 in autistic spectrum disorders. Prostaglandins Leukot Essent Fatty Acids 2004;71(4):201–4.
38. Meguid NA, Atta HM, Gouda AS, et al. Role of polyunsaturated fatty acids in the management of Egyptian children with autism. Clin Biochem 2008;41(13): 1044–8.
39. Vancassel S, Durand G, Barthelemy C, et al. Plasma fatty acid levels in autistic children. Prostaglandins Leukot Essent Fatty Acids 2001;65(1):1–7.
40. Meiri G, Bichovsky Y, Belmaker RH. Omega 3 fatty acid treatment in autism. J Child Adolesc Psychopharmacol 2009;19(4):449–51.
41. Johnson CR, Handen BL, ZImmer M, et al. Polyunsaturated fatty acid supplementation in young children with autism. J Dev Phys Disabil 2010;22(1):1–10.
42. Amminger GP, Berger GE, Schafer MR, et al. Omega-3 fatty acids supplementation in children with autism: a double-blind randomized, placebo-controlled pilot study. Biol Psychiatry 2007;61(4):551–3.

43. Bent S, Bertoglio K, Ashwood P, et al. A pilot randomized controlled trial of omega-3 fatty acids for autism spectrum disorder. J Autism Dev Disord 2011; 41(5):545–54.
44. Bloch MH, Qawasmi A. Omega-3 fatty acid supplementation for the treatment of children with attention-deficit/hyperactivity disorder symptomatology: systematic review and meta-analysis. J Am Acad Child Adolesc Psychiatry 2011; 50(10):991–1000.
45. Gillies D, Sinn J, Lad SS, et al. Polyunsaturated fatty acids (PUFA) for attention deficit hyperactivity disorder (ADHD) in children and adolescents. Cochrane Database Syst Rev 2012;(7):CD007986.
46. Bertoglio K, Jill James S, Deprey L, et al. Pilot study of the effect of methyl B12 treatment on behavioral and biomarker measures in children with autism. J Altern Complement Med 2010;16(5):555–60.
47. Hardan AY, Fung LK, Libove RA, et al. A randomized controlled pilot trial of oral N-acetylcysteine in children with autism. Biol Psychiatry 2012;71(11):956–61 PMID:22342106.
48. Adams JB, Audhya T, McDonough-Means S, et al. Effect of a vitamin/mineral supplement on children and adults with autism. BMC Pediatr 2011;11:111.
49. Munasinghe SA, Oliff C, Finn J, et al. Digestive enzyme supplementation for autism spectrum disorders: a double-blind randomized controlled trial. J Autism Dev Disord 2010;40(9):1131–8.
50. Adams JB, Audhya T, McDonough-Means S, et al. Nutritional and metabolic status of children with autism vs. neurotypical children, and the association with autism severity. Nutr Metab (Lond) 2011;8(1):34.
51. Mehl-Madrona L, Leung B, Kennedy C, et al. Micronutrients versus standard medication management in autism: a naturalistic case-control study. J Child Adolesc Psychopharmacol 2010;20(2):95–103.
52. Adams JB, Holloway C. Pilot study of a moderate dose multivitamin/mineral supplement for children with autistic spectrum disorder. J Altern Complement Med 2004;10(6):1033–9.
53. Gupta S. Treatment of children with autism with intravenous immunoglobulin. J Child Neurol 1999;14(3):203–5.
54. Adams JB, Baral M, Geis E, et al. Safety and efficacy of oral DMSA therapy for children with autism spectrum disorders: part A–medical results. BMC Clin Pharmacol 2009;9:16.
55. Adams JB, Baral M, Geis E, et al. Safety and efficacy of oral DMSA therapy for children with autism spectrum disorders: part B - behavioral results. BMC Clin Pharmacol 2009;9:17.

Learning and Cognitive Disorders
Multidiscipline Treatment Approaches

Anil Chacko, PhD[a,b,c,*], Jodi Uderman, BA[a], Nicole Feirsen, BA[a],
Anne-Claude Bedard, PhD[b], David Marks, PhD[c]

KEYWORDS

- Youth • Children • Adolescents • Learning disorders • Working memory
- Auditory processing disorders • Treatment • Intervention

KEY POINTS

- Numerous interventions with varying evidence bases exist for the treatment of learning and cognitive disorders.
- There are clear evidence-based interventions for reading disorders (eg, peer-assisted learning strategies) and disorder of written expression (eg, self-regulated strategy development).
- There is emerging evidence suggesting that certain intervention approaches (eg, fact-retrieval intervention, schema-based instruction, mnemonic strategy instruction, cognitive strategy instruction) may be beneficial for mathematics disorder, but will require more rigorous evaluation.
- A concrete-to-representational-to-abstract strategy for the treatment of mathematics disorder has good evidence for middle-school and high-school students.
- Although several commercially available interventions exist for the treatment of auditory processing disorder and poor working memory, review of the existing literature suggests caution in using these treatments.

INTRODUCTION

Learning and cognitive disorders affect a substantial number of youth, resulting in considerable concurrent impairment and diminishing the potential for successful long-term academic and social functioning of affected youth. Given these issues,

Disclosures: The authors have no disclosures to report.
[a] Department of Psychology, The Graduate School and University Center, Queens College, City University of New York (CUNY), 65-30 Kissena Boulevard, Flushing, NY 11367, USA; [b] Department of Psychiatry, The Mount Sinai School of Medicine, 1468 Madison Avenue, New York, NY 10029, USA; [c] Department of Child and Adolescent Psychiatry, New York University School of Medicine, One Park Avenue, 7th Floor, New York, NY 10016, USA
* Corresponding author. Department of Psychology, The Graduate School and University Center, Queens College, City University of New York (CUNY), 65-30 Kissena Boulevard, Flushing, NY 11367.
E-mail address: anil.chacko@qc.cuny.edu

Child Adolesc Psychiatric Clin N Am 22 (2013) 457–477
http://dx.doi.org/10.1016/j.chc.2013.03.006
1056-4993/13/$ – see front matter © 2013 Elsevier Inc. All rights reserved.

childpsych.theclinics.com

considerable investment has been made in developing and evaluating treatments to address these problems. A comprehensive review of all interventions focused on various learning and cognitive disorders is well beyond the scope of this article; the authors focus instead on a select review of interventions that are commonly used to address reading disorder, mathematics disorder, disorder of written expression, poor working memory, and auditory processing disorder. As the reader will glean from this review, there are numerous treatments, many publicly available, for addressing these issues. Although several interventions are well established for certain disorders, there are several that require considerably more rigorous evaluation. **Table 1** summarizes the interventions reviewed herein, and **Table 2** recaps the authors' opinions regarding the value of these interventions for the various disorders.

READING DISORDERS

Reading disorders are neurobiological conditions with deficient phonologic coding. Subsequently, interventions aimed at this underlying etiology have been the most efficacious. Although many different remediation programs exist, there is no one "magic" program identified in the literature[1]; rather, programs that encompass shared, critical components are recommended.[1,2] Essential elements of such interventions include individualization, feedback and guidance, ongoing assessment, and regular ongoing practice.[3] Programs should be highly structured and intensive, and should include explicit reading instruction. Content should be organized in a hierarchical manner, starting with phonemic awareness, sound-symbol association, phonics, awareness of rhyme, and word segmentation. Phonemic awareness involves the ability of a listener to be able to hear, identify, and manipulate phonemes, the smallest units of sound that can differentiate meaning. Separating the spoken word "cat" into 3 distinct phonemes, k/, /æ/, and /t/, requires phonemic awareness. As children develop, instruction should advance to fluency training, vocabulary, and comprehension, then to syllable instruction, morphology, memorizing sight words, spelling, syntax, and semantics.[4] In particular, a multisensory, small-group approach that focuses on applying phonemic awareness skills and phonemic manipulation, particularly with letters (vs sounds) is most commonly recommended.[2,5]

Using curricula with many of these components, for younger children (k to first grade), small-group instruction (2–3:1) that occurs 4 to 5 times a week that includes phonologic awareness, letter knowledge, and explicit phonics is recommended.[2] Younger children have the best outcome using this methodology, often with long-term gains. For older children, improved outcomes have been achieved with 1-on-1 instruction, with more intensive work for a longer duration in comparison with younger youth. In general, reading comprehension appears to be most directly affected by intervention, with less improvement observed in spelling and fluency.

The Orton-Gillingham approach has been used since the 1930s for reading intervention, and many commercial remediation programs based on this approach are available (eg, the Wilson Reading System, Project Read, Alphabetic Phonics, the Herman method, the Slingerland method, Language!, and the Spalding method). The Orton-Gillingham approach is a multisensory, sequential, phonics-based system that focuses on basic word formation before whole meanings. Few of the commercial programs, however, have been tested in rigorous, randomized controlled trials.[5] School-based programs that have been more widely studied include Lindamood phoneme sequencing (LiPS),[6] Fast ForWord (FFW),[7] and Peer-assisted learning strategies (PALS).[8] Although many other programs exist, the literature on their evaluation is scarce.[9–11]

Table 1
Overview of select treatments and approaches for learning and cognitive disorders

Area	Intervention/Approach	Summary	Basis in Youth	Modified USPSTF System (Quality of Evidence/Strength of Recommendation)
Reading disorder	Orton-Gillingham approach	Multisensory, sequential, phonics-based system that focuses on basic word formation	Adequate RCTs	Good/Recommended
	Lindamood phoneme sequencing	Multisensory, bottom-up, explicit approach for developing phonemic awareness and phonemic decoding skills with minimal text instruction	Adequate RCTs	Fair/Neutral
	Fast ForWord	Computer-based program that consists of a series of adaptive, interactive exercises that use acoustically processed speech and speech sounds	Adequate RCTs	Good/Neutral
	Peer-assisted learning strategies	Peer-tutoring, repeated reading, and paragraph summary with corrective feedback	Adequate RCTs	Good/Strongly recommended
	RAVE-O	Multicomponent program to address both overt reading behaviors like word recognition skills and comprehension, and underlying components	Adequate RCTs	Good/Strongly Recommended
	PHAST	Comprehensive intervention focused on developing word decoding skills and decoding strategies	Adequate RCTs	Good/Strongly Recommended

(continued on next page)

Table 1
(continued)

Area	Intervention/Approach	Summary	Basis in Youth	Modified USPSTF System (Quality of Evidence/Strength of Recommendation)
Mathematics disorder	Fact retrieval intervention	Programs comprise computer-based instruction, math fact flash card practice sessions, and fact review with individualized feedback	Uncontrolled designs	Fair/Recommended
	Concrete-to-representational-to-abstract	Comprises 3 primary sequenced components: the use of physical manipulations of concrete objects, followed by the use of graphic representations of these concrete objects, followed by the teaching of abstract thinking specifically geared toward problem solving	Adequate RCTs	Good/Strong recommendation for older youth
	Cognitive strategy instruction	Goals of this type of intervention are to automatize the cognitive processes critical to problem solving and to encourage self-regulation	Uncontrolled studies	Fair/Recommended
	Mnemonic strategy	Teaching students to apply mnemonic devices to mathematical operations as a heuristic technique	Uncontrolled studies and RCT	Fair/Recommended
	Schema-based instruction	Direct instruction on how to schematically interpret word problems	Uncontrolled studies	Fair/Recommended

Disorder of written expression	Strategies for planning/drafting	Supporting students to use discrete planning and drafting procedures	Adequate RCTs	Good/Strongly Recommended
	Strategies for editing	Supporting students to use discrete planning and drafting procedures	Uncontrolled studies	Fair/Recommended
	Goal setting	Identifying goals for writing quantity/quality with rewards for goal attainment	Uncontrolled studies	Fair/Recommended
	Word processing	Using word-processing features to support editing of text	Uncontrolled studies	Fair/Recommended
Low working memory	Cogmed working memory training	Computerized adaptive training of storage and manipulation of verbal and nonverbal working memory components	Multiple RCTs	Good/Neutral
Auditory processing disorder	Auditory integration training	Focuses on improving hearing distortions and hearing hypo/hypersensitivity	One RCT; uncontrolled studies	Poor/Recommend against
	Tomatis method	Focuses on improving auditory functioning through stimulation	Uncontrolled study	Poor/Insufficient evidence to recommend for or against
	Earobics	Comprehensive computer-based program for training phonologic awareness and auditory language-processing skills	Adequate RCTs	Good/Neutral
	Fact ForWord	Adaptive intervention that uses modified sounds (speech and nonspeech) to train temporal processing, speech perception, and language comprehension skills	Adequate RCTs	Good/Neutral

Quality of evidence: good (strong quality), fair (mixed quality), no data (no empirical data available to make recommendation), poor (sufficiently weak data to support intervention). Strength of the evidence is graded as strongly recommends, recommends, no recommendation for or against, recommends against, or insufficient evidence to recommend for or against.

Abbreviations: RCT, randomized controlled trial; USPSTF, US Preventive Services Task Force.

Table 2
Treatment evaluation: the authors' personal opinion

Intervention/Approach	Outcomes	Modified USPSTF System (Quality of Evidence/Strength of Recommendation)	Opinion
Orton-Gillingham approach	Reading	Good/Recommended	General approach focused on phonologic processing/awareness, word analysis, reading fluency, and reading comprehension is useful
Lindamood phoneme sequencing	Reading	Fair/No Recommendation for or against	Less intensive interventions found to be as useful
Fast ForWord	Reading	Good/No Recommendation for or against	Less intensive interventions are found to be as useful. Likely not beneficial
Peer-assisted learning strategies	Reading	Good/Strongly recommended	Good to use; requires minimal training; small adaptations to classroom must be made to implement this
RAVE-O	Reading	Good/Strongly recommended	Good to use, particularly for children with significant reading difficulties
PHAST	Reading	Good/Strongly Recommended	Good to use, and can be integrated into classroom
Fact retrieval intervention	Math	Fair/Recommended	Easy to implement but used as a second-line intervention
Concrete-to-representational-to-abstract	Math	Good/Strong recommendation for older youth	Strong support for use but may be more challenging for younger youth
Cognitive strategy instruction	Math	Fair/Recommended	More investment from teacher to implement effectively; may be more challenging for younger youth

Mnemonic strategy	Math	Fair/Recommended	Easy to implement and can be used for all ages
Schema-based instruction	Math	Fair/Recommended	More investment from teacher to implement effectively; may be more challenging for younger youth
Strategies for planning/drafting	Written expression	Good/Strongly Recommended	More investment from teacher to implement effectively; strongly recommended
Strategies for editing	Written expression	Fair/Recommended	More investment from teacher to implement effectively
Goal setting	Written expression	Fair/Recommended	Simple strategy and should have benefits if applied broadly (for entire classroom)
Word processing	Written expression	Fair/Recommended	Increased use of computers in classrooms will allow for more use of this method. Can and should be used
Cogmed working memory training	Poor working memory	Good/No recommendation for or against	Considerable effort and compliance needed to attain benefits. Some questions as to whether intervention has impact on broader assessment of working memory
Auditory integration training	Auditory processing	Poor/Recommend against	Costs and supportive data likely prohibit the use of intervention
Tomatis method	Auditory processing	Poor/Insufficient evidence to recommend for or against	Costs and supportive data likely prohibit the use of intervention
Earobics	Auditory processing	Good/No recommendation for or against	Unclear clinical implications
Fact ForWord	Auditory processing	Good/No recommendation for or against	Unclear clinical implications

LiPS is a multisensory, bottom-up, explicit approach for developing phonemic awareness and phonemic decoding skills with minimal text instruction. FFW is a computer-based program that consists of a series of adaptive, interactive exercises that use acoustically processed speech and speech sounds. PALS uses peer tutoring, repeated reading, and paragraph summary, with corrective feedback. These interventions have been evaluated in controlled trials, primarily in school-age children from diverse socioeconomic backgrounds in various settings (eg, school, summer camps). However, the methods of implementation for these interventions have varied considerably across studies.[8,12–18]

Research on LiPS has revealed that children improve in alphabetics and reading fluency, with no effects on reading comprehension.[13,14] These studies reported that alternative interventions that shared critical components with LiPS (eg, phonemic awareness and decoding, using explicit, systematic instruction) but differed in delivery were also effective. This finding suggests that teachers implementing core principles of effective practice, rather than LiPS per se, can expect benefits on reading outcomes. Of note, 40% of the children across these interventions were no longer in special education classrooms at follow-up; however, only about half sustained gains and one-quarter lost gains over a 2-year period.[14] Effect size (ES) data on primary outcomes of focus in these studies have considerable variability (ES = 0.12–0.54).

Research suggests that overall, the intensive training and cost necessary for implementing FFW is not warranted (see also the section on FFW for auditory processing disorder). For example, although one study found improvements in phonemic awareness after FFW, gains were similar to those of the comparison group, which was a less intensive Orton-Gillingham program.[12] A second study found significant gains in nonword reading, word identification, passage comprehension, receptive and expressive language, and rapid naming after FFW; however, only nonword reading outcomes improved enough to be considered clinically meaningful.[16] ES data on primary outcomes of focus in these studies range from no effect to a small positive effect (ES = 0.12–0.32).

Results from rigorous studies on PALS indicate positive effects on reading fluency and reading comprehension, relative to comparison groups (eg, typical instruction).[19,20] In an evaluation of the PALS literature, What Works Clearinghouse calculated large enough effect sizes for reading fluency and reading comprehension to declare a "substantial, positive effect" in these domains.[21] ES data on primary outcomes of focus in these studies are large (ES >0.80).

Most recently, 2 comprehensive reading interventions have been studied that suggest clear benefits for youth with reading impairments. RAVE-O (http://ase.tufts.edu/crlr/RAVE-O/) addresses both overt reading behaviors, such as word-recognition skills and comprehension, and underlying components (eg, visual scanning, lexical retrieval). RAVE-O simultaneously addresses the need for automaticity in key systems related to reading (eg, phonologic and morphologic systems) as well as the importance of teaching explicit connections among these systems. The goal throughout is to teach systematic, theoretical principles that underlie fluency and decoding through explicit instruction in skills underlying fluency and comprehension; imaginative, whimsy-filled opportunities for practice; and a set of strategies that embolden discouraged children to look at written language through new eyes. PHAST (http://www.sickkids.ca/LDRP/Empower-Reading/Program-description/index.html) is a comprehensive intervention focused on developing word-decoding skills and decoding strategies. Studies have documented effects for both of these interventions across reading and language outcomes, and are highly recommended interventions for struggling readers.

It should also be noted that vision-based therapies are advertised as remedying reading disabilities as well (eg, eye exercises, behavioral vision therapy, or special tinted filters or lenses). The American Academy of Pediatrics, however, noted that vision therapies are not supported by sound research, and are therefore not recommended as evidence-based treatments.[22] Although vision may interfere with learning to read, it is not considered to be the primary cause of impairment.

MATHEMATICS DISORDER

Math-related learning disorders (MLD) are present in approximately 5% to 8% of students.[23] These children tend to experience difficulty with procedural operations, working memory, conceptual understanding of numbers, problem-solving strategies, and organizing information,[24] so that they children frequently fall behind in school. However, given the diverse symptomatology and the lack of a standardized diagnostic tool, there does not currently appear to be one gold-standard intervention.

One type of MLD treatment with some empirical support is known broadly as fact retrieval intervention.[25–28] This type of program is founded on the theory that quickly and efficiently accessing learned number combinations is a critical step in rudimentary mathematics. Thus, if children have deficits in this automatized retrieval process, they will be unable to achieve proficient, grade-appropriate math skills. These interventions (eg, Hasselbring, Goin, and Bransford's "Fast Facts") are computer-based instructional tools centered on imparting fact-retrieval strategies. Most programs comprise computer-based instruction, math-fact flash-card practice sessions, and fact review with individualized feedback. Although multiple studies have tested this type of intervention, methodological limitations (ie, no control group, lack of random assignment, and so forth) limit conclusions that can be drawn regarding the efficacy of this approach. ES data on primary outcomes of focus in these studies range from a small to moderate effect (ES = 0.23–0.58).

Concrete-to-representational-to-abstract (CRA) comprises 3 primary sequenced components: the use of physical manipulations of concrete objects, followed by the use of graphic representations of these concrete objects, followed by the teaching of abstract thinking specifically geared toward problem solving.[29] The CRA model is categorized as a multisensory approach because it integrates visual, auditory, kinesthetic, and tactile interactions with content through the direct handling of objects and matching of graphic designs. CRA principles have been used to help students with MLD learn various mathematical operations including word problems,[30] fractions,[31] linear functions,[32] and algebra,[29] but it has almost exclusively been used in middle-school and high-school settings. ES data on primary outcomes of focus in these studies range from a small to moderate effect (ES = 0.21–0.52).

Cognitive strategy instruction (eg, "Solve It!"[33]) focuses on the planning and execution of cognitive tasks.[34] The overriding goals of this type of intervention are to automate the cognitive processes critical to problem solving and to encourage self-regulation (namely, self-instruction, self-questioning, and self-monitoring) during mathematical operations. Cognitive strategy instruction has been tested in students with learning disorders.[33] Overall this technique appears to show great promise, but will require further rigorous evaluation as regards improving the math skills of children with MLD.

Mnemonic strategy instruction targets teaching students to apply mnemonic devices to mathematical operations as a heuristic technique. For example, one model, LAP Fractions,[35] instructs children to "look at the sign and denominator, ask yourself the question: will the smallest denominator divide into the largest denominator an even number of times, Pick your fraction type," to assist in fraction-related problems. Another variation of this type of intervention assigns stories and characters to different mathematical operations to assist in the memorization of difficult rules and procedures.[36] Again, the results of this category of intervention are promising, but further research should be completed to assess generalizability across ages and math levels.

Schema-based instruction, which has received empirical support,[37–39] includes direct instruction on how to schematically interpret word problems (eg, identify the operation being asked, then use schema-based reasoning and logic to organize problem-solving efforts). Theoretically, proficient problem solvers create mental representations of the problem schema to solve the question accurately. These schemas can then be generalized to structurally similar prompts, which should increase efficacy and decrease the cognitive load required to complete the computation. Although this technique has garnered some empirical support, many of the studies included a small number of participants, were conducted by the same research group, and only focused on very specific types of mathematical problems. ES data on primary outcomes of focus in these studies range from a small to moderate effect (ES = 0.38–0.61). Future research should attempt to replicate the results of these initial trials.

DISORDER OF WRITTEN EXPRESSION

Disorder of written expression is a learning disorder in which an individual's writing ability is significantly below the expected range given the person's chronologic age, intelligence, and age-appropriate education. Writing skills must also result in significant impairment in academic achievement or activities of daily living that require the composition of written texts. Numerous interventions to improve writing skills of youth affected with disorder of written expression have been identified, and have resulted in significant benefits for affected youth.

Strategy instruction methods have been evaluated to improve various aspects of writing skills in youth with disorder of written expression. Methods that focus on teaching strategies for planning/drafting specific types of text, principally using self-regulated strategy development,[40] have received considerable empirical support in improving structural elements of composition, writing productivity, and writing quality. These improvements are generally maintained over time and are generalized beyond trained content. Methods for teaching strategies for editing have also been conducted, with findings generally supporting the effects of this strategy on error detection. To date, strategies for planning/drafting have the most robust empirical support[40–42] for youth with disorder for written expression. A recent meta-analysis[43] also suggests that this strategy offers considerable promise for youth with primary disabilities other than learning disorders (eg, attention-deficit/hyperactivity disorder, emotional or behavioral disorders). ES data on primary outcomes of focus in these studies range from a moderate to large effect (ES = 0.57–1.1).

A secondary set of methods have also been used, and have demonstrated significant benefit in improving various aspects of writing skills.[40–42] For example, establishing specific and clear goals (ie, goal setting) improves the quality of text and writing productivity. Studies have used goal setting in various ways, including having students self-monitor goals with public recognition for achieving a goal to teachers establishing writing goals and providing direct feedback on goal achievement. Studies suggest benefits of goal setting on increasing productivity (number of words written, number or percentage of writing assignments completed). In addition, students' writing appears to derive considerable benefit from the use of word processing. Studies that have focused on using word processing in lieu of handwriting or word processing with prompts to use editing features of the word-processing programs have demonstrated benefits with respect to increasing writing productivity. Finally, teaching students how best to write different types of sentences and how to combine simpler sentences into more complex sentences have also demonstrated a positive impact on the number of complete sentences produced.

Several interventions, primarily supported through single-subject research designs, also suggest benefits for students with writing difficulties. For example, in a meta-analysis, benefit was reported for reinforcing students for writing productivity, as well as teaching strategies for editing text and strategies for constructing paragraphs.[41] More rigorous evaluations are necessary to provide further support for these interventions.

WORKING MEMORY

Working memory, once considered a fixed attribute, is now considered malleable and, importantly, improvable through direct intervention. This malleability is important, as working memory is considered a core executive function that is related to a host of important outcomes for individuals, including academic and professional success. The premise is that if working memory can be improved, there will be benefits across key outcomes (eg, attention) that are critical for long-term adjustment in youth.

Over the past decade there has been an explosion of commercial and scientific interest in developing and evaluating interventions that improve working memory in both children and adults. For instance, MindSparke, Lumosity, Jungle Memory, Growing with Timocco, and Play Attention are now readily available for commercial use.[44] Unfortunately, commercial development has far outpaced high-quality experimental evaluation of these interventions. For some interventions, practically no rigorous studies published in peer-reviewed outlets have been conducted. As such, it is impossible to state anything more than that these remain untested interventions. To date, Cogmed working memory training (CWMT) has stood out as a leader in the working-memory training movement, given the number of independent empirical studies of CWMT. A review of CWMT offers an opportunity to objectively critique working-memory training interventions.

Briefly, CWMT is a computerized training program designed to effectively increase working-memory capacity over a 5-week training period through targeting both storage and manipulation of verbal and nonverbal working-memory components. Training takes place in approximately 30- to 45-minute increments over 5 days per week (25 training days in total). CWMT trials are individualized/titrated to the capacity of the individual using an adaptive, staircase design that adjusts the difficulty of the program on a trial-by-trial basis; that is, correct trials are followed by successive trials with heightened working-memory demands, whereas incorrect trials result in subsequent trials with diminished working-memory load. Support for implementation is provided by a CWMT training aide (usually a parent) and a certified CWMT coach, who solves implementation problems with the trainee and training aide on a weekly basis.

Studies across children and adults in clinical (eg, youth with attention-deficit/hyperactivity disorder, learning disorders, stroke patients, individuals with acquired brain injury) and typically developing populations using several treatment designs (eg, open clinical trials, randomized clinical trials) with various comparison conditions (eg, wait-list control, attention-control) have documented the effects of CWMT. For example, CWMT has been shown to improve working memory,[45,46] brain activity,[47] and attention.[46,48,49] ES data on primary outcomes of focus in these studies range from a moderate to large effect (ES = 0.52–1.12).

More recently, however, considerable concerns have been raised regarding the literature on CWMT specifically,[50–53] as well as caution regarding the effusive claims made by cognitive training programs in general.[44,54] For instance, there have been inconsistent findings in the literature regarding the results of CWMT between studies[46,55] as well as within studies.[56] Some have suggested that there is poor transfer of training from trained working-memory tasks to untrained working-memory tasks, and further downstream to more complex tasks (eg, reasoning and attention).[50] However, the extant data regarding specific effects of CWMT on specific working-memory outcomes suggest some benefit, although further research is needed.

AUDITORY PROCESSING DISORDER

Youth with auditory processing disorder (APD) have significant difficulties in identifying, discriminating, ordering, grouping, or localizing sounds. APD appears to be very common in youth with specific reading disorders or specific language impairment, with some studies suggesting that youth with attention-deficit/hyperactivity disorder or autism also suffer from APD. Although identified decades ago, APD has only recently received consideration as a diagnostic entity.[57] Likewise, the treatment of APD has received more attention over the past decade, with several empirical studies evaluating a variety of treatments.

Treatments for APD have taken various forms and have differed as regards the conceptual focus of the treatment. For instance, auditory treatments manipulate auditory components of speech and nonspeech language (eg, FFW), whereas language treatments manipulate language form, content, and use (eg, Earobics).[58] Environmental modification (eg, preferential seating; hearing aids) and compensatory strategies (eg, memory and attention strategies) have also been used to support youth with APD. Herein the treatment literature on auditory integration training (AIT), Tomatis, Earobics, and FFW is discussed, given the use of these interventions in clinical practice.

AIT focuses on improving hearing distortions and hearing hyposensitivity/hypersensitivity, which impair an individual's attention, comprehension and, therefore, learning. AIT involves multisession sound therapy whereby individuals use headphones to listen to modulated music from an AIT device to normalize hearing responses. AIT has been used as a treatment for various clinical disorders (eg, autism, attention-deficit/hyperactivity disorder) as well as for individuals with APD across the life span. Despite its long history, there have been very few rigorous evaluations of AIT for the treatment of APD. In fact, the only study that has been conducted on school-age youth with APD or language disorders suggests no benefit of AIT.[59] This study reported the effects of AIT relative to a control condition on various behavioral and physiologic outcomes, and found no differential benefit of AIT on these outcomes. Several other studies have been conducted on AIT, but lack the experimental rigor needed to be able to support the utility of AIT for treating youth with APD and/or language disorders. There is thus no clear empirical justification for AIT in the treatment of APD.

The Tomatis method, developed in the 1950s, aims to more efficiently transmit and process acoustic sensory messages via the stimulation of muscles in the ear through the use of specialized auditory equipment that is calibrated to the profile of the user. Despite the use of the Tomatis method for the treatment of APD (as well as other disorders including language disorders, emotion disorder, attention disorders, and autism spectrum disorders) over several decades and its use in practice settings internationally, few studies have systematically evaluated the benefits of this method. A meta-analysis[60] found no effect on auditory-related outcomes across studies using the Tomatis method. More recently, Ross-Swain,[61] who evaluated retrospective reports of individuals between the ages of 4 and 19 years who completed the Tomatis method, found significant benefits of the method on auditory memory, sequencing, discrimination, and cohesion. This study is limited in that it used a nonrandomized retrospective design of selected patients who completed the 90-hour Tomatis method. These patients were not assessed for APD but had features commonly associated with APD. Given the current state of the literature, further empirical evaluation is needed before one can recommend the Tomatis method for the treatment of APD.

Earobics is a comprehensive computer-based program used to improve phonologic awareness and auditory language-processing skills. Few studies have been conducted on Earobics for the treatment of APD,[62–64] and they have had mixed findings. For instance, several studies[62–64] reported positive training effects of Earobics on phonologic awareness skills and neurophysiologic factors related to auditory processing, but did not find effects on reading and spelling outcomes. One study, using a series of case studies, found mixed benefits of Earobics on reading and spelling across study participants.[65] Another report evaluated the effects of Earobics in a comparison with other treatment methods, and found no significant benefit of Earobics on language outcomes.[15] Collectively the handful of studies on Earobics have mixed findings, which suggest caution and further exploration of this therapy as a potential intervention for youth with APD and/or language disorders.

FFW is an adaptive intervention that uses modified sounds (speech and nonspeech) to train temporal processing, speech perception, and language comprehension skills. To date, this intervention has undergone the most extensive empirical investigation, with more than 20 studies evaluating FFW as an intervention for APD and/or language disorders. Collectively, findings across these studies have been mixed. For instance, some exploratory studies have documented significant improvements in auditory measures[65–67] and language outcomes.[68,69] However, more methodologically rigorous studies have found no specific effect of FFW on auditory outcomes or language outcomes,[15,58,70,71] with ES in the zero to small effect range (ES = 0.08–0.23).

SUMMARY
Clinical Implications

When predicting treatment response in youth with reading disorders, baseline phonologic awareness and rapid naming ability have consistently emerged as important factors for successful outcomes.[72] However, there is also evidence to suggest that reading outcomes have multiple determinants and that other, broader neurocognitive factors should be included in this discussion. Indeed, baseline visual, verbal, and memory processes have also been shown to be important predictors, in addition to phonologic awareness and rapid naming.[73] This evidence suggests that those with poor baseline functioning in other cognitive domains not traditionally associated with reading outcome may have little to no treatment response, so that traditional treatments may not be an appropriate recommendation. As such, it would be important to have a more comprehensive evaluation of the child's neurocognitive functioning when planning treatment, to predict treatment response to traditional interventions and to more appropriately individualize treatment. Lastly, when considering treatment recommendations it would also be important to correctly identify the underlying cause of the reading difficulty. For instance, although dyslexia is most widely studied, there are other reading disorders that have distinct neurobiological underpinnings,[74] which therefore may have different treatment considerations. For instance, youth may also have a specific comprehension deficit, with intact word-level abilities. Evidence suggests that these youth may have difficulty accessing lexical-semantic representations during word recognition.[74] It is therefore important to keep in mind that other causes exist and that the correct identification of reading difficulty is important in appropriately individualizing treatment.

In light of the extant literature, some general implications for the treatment of reading disorders, include the use of intensive, explicit training with critical elements including individualization, feedback and guidance, ongoing assessment, and regular ongoing practice. Explicit reading instruction organized in a hierarchical manner starting with phonemic awareness and sound-symbol association is efficacious, with considerable latitude regarding delivery. However, specific commercially available programs are often costly and difficult to implement, and require trained specialists; this is often unfeasible for many school-based or home-based programs. By contrast, there is empirical support that PALS has substantial effects on multiple reading domains while being relatively easy to implement. In terms of potential costs for clinicians and parents interested in using interventions for reading disorder, it is cost-effective to opt for individual or small-group learning that is focused on explicit and intensive treatments. Commercially available programs will clearly be more costly, but there are few conclusive data suggesting that these improve outcomes. The cost of PALS is also minimal and is a one-time cost; once the material is purchased it can be subsequently used in the classroom without additional costs. Both RAVE-O and PHAST incorporate multiple, evidence-based methods to improve reading and language, and have demonstrated significant benefits for struggling readers, Given the strong data supporting PALS, RAVE-O, and PHAST, and the relatively minimal costs, these are interventions that are highly recommended for school-based use.

There is a growing recognition that youth who present with mathematics disorders suffer from various and multiple deficits (eg, poor math facts, poor calculation fluency[24,75]), and often also have underlying broad deficits in working memory, which compounds difficulties in math because children are required to use increasing levels of working memory when completing more advanced mathematics calculations.[75] As such, it is important to go beyond standardized assessments of math achievement tests to include more specific evaluation of math deficits (facts, skills, and so forth) to provide personalized approaches to targeting the specific math deficits that a child may suffer from. At present, although there are numerous interventions and approaches for treating mathematics disorder, it seems that interventions comprising repeated practice trials and concrete, easily relatable examples, instructions, or strategies have garnered the most empirical support. It also appears that interventions should target the most basic elements of a given skill to ensure that children are learning and understanding the principles underlying the mathematical operations. This extra support should be provided to children as early as possible to prevent them from falling farther behind.

There is substantial evidence from numerous studies that methods focused on teaching strategies for planning/drafting specific types of text have considerable empirical support for addressing difficulties with written expression. In particular, self-regulated strategy development appears to be a first-line intervention for treating writing skills. Likewise, there appears to be considerable support for other interventions (eg, goal setting, use of word processing). These interventions, although less effective, are beneficial. Given the relative simplicity of goal setting and the increasing use of word processing in schools, these interventions should be consistently made use of, preferably along with strategies for planning/drafting texts. The costs of the reviewed treatments for MLD are minimal, and these methods are likely good practice for supporting math learning in youth, although some more cognitively complex interventions may be more challenging for younger youth.

Although there has been considerable interest and investment in the development of treatments for improving working memory, there is considerable debate regarding the efficacy of such approaches. Of importance is that although there are numerous commercially available interventions for improving working memory, there have been limited, if any, rigorous and independently conducted evaluations to test the claims of these interventions. Given the numerous conceptual issues and methodological limitations of CWMT, a firm conclusion regarding the benefits of CWMT cannot be made. However, there appears to be some stronger support for CWMT on core working-memory components that are "trained" during treatment, with more concern about the transfer of these abilities to nontrained tasks. More rigorous evaluation is clearly needed. The cost of CWMT may be substantial, as these are provided directly by a CWMT-certified practitioner (usually a physician or psychologist). This intervention may be cost-prohibitive for families with fewer financial resources.

Collectively, there is great variability in the number and methodological rigor of studies that have evaluated AIT, the Tomatis method, Earobics, and FFW for the treatment of APD. In general, there is limited evidence supporting Earobics and FFW, with no compelling evidence supporting AIT or the Tomatis method as an intervention for APD or related problems of language and academic performance. The conclusions presented herein suggest that clinicians should conduct a careful assessment for APD, with accompanying assessments focused on problems with language, reading, and academic achievement. Evidence-based treatments (some of which are reviewed herein) should target these accompanying problems as the first line of therapy. There should be close monitoring of progress with these interventions to determine ongoing response to treatment. If there appears to be little improvement despite high-quality implementation of these interventions, an intervention focused on treating identified auditory processing issues may be warranted. This approach will also require ongoing monitoring of the impact of an APD treatment, not only on auditory outcomes but also on language, reading, and academic performance. Similar to CWMT, many of these interventions are commercially packaged and only available through a certified provider. However, given the status of the evidence for these interventions in treating APD, there is little rationale for the use of these interventions.

Research Implications

Multiple research implications derive from this review. First, there is a great need to understand how characteristics of youth and their contexts (eg, family, classroom) moderate treatment response. Knowing for whom and under what contexts a well-supported intervention is more or less effective has clear implications for practice. These types of studies are clearly necessary for treatments that have robust empirical support. Similarly, many interventions (eg, FFW) reviewed herein are multifaceted, although it is unclear as to which components of these interventions are having a direct impact on outcomes. Research directed at understanding the underlying mechanisms of how a particular treatment affects key outcomes is clearly needed to develop more parsimonious treatments. The resulting refined and simplified treatments and approaches are likely to be more closely adhered to, and will allow for the delivery of a more potent dose of the active ingredients, which should directly result in improved outcomes.

There are multiple interventions reviewed herein that offer promise but have been inadequately studied (eg, reinforcing students for writing productivity, schema-based instruction for math). More rigorous studies must be conducted with these interventions, as there is a need to identify alternative approaches to the treatment of learning and cognitive disorders given patient and provider preferences, heterogeneity in response to treatment, and moderators of treatment response. Having a robust armamentarium of evidence-based treatments will allow for greater tailoring of treatment.

Of the areas reviewed herein, the treatment of poor working memory (and interventions to enhance neurocognitive functioning in general) is likely the most promising line of future empirical investigation. Given the importance of working memory, there needs to be continued investment in further refining CWMT (as well as other working-memory interventions). Such efforts are an increasing focus of second-generation studies.[76] More generally, with the advances gained through the ever-growing literature on neuroscience, we are discovering how the brain is affected in youth with learning and cognitive disorders, and are increasingly better able to develop interventions that more precisely target these underlying deficits and mechanisms. There is no simple translation of findings from basic science into psychosocial treatment, but there is great potential to provide tailored and perhaps more effective treatment through this line of empirical inquiry.

Before closing, it is beneficial to briefly discuss the emerging data on the neurobiological underpinning of learning disorders (ie, reading and mathematics disorders), whereby data may begin to better inform the potential targets for treatment and provide more personalized treatment regimes. For reading disorders,[77] there has been increasing recognition that there is an underactivation of left hemisphere temporoparietal regions that may affect phonologic processing and underactivation of the left hemisphere occipitotemporal region, which is believed to be important for word recognition. There is also evidence that implicates white-matter disruption in the left hemisphere perisylvian regions. In mathematics learning disorders,[78] there is an interrelationship between the occipitotemporal lobe (fusiform gyrus), parietal lobe (intraparietal sulcus and angular gyrus), and frontal lobe (prefrontal cortex), which is responsible for potential difficulties in mathematics. For instance, the occipitotemporal and parietal lobes are required for mapping digits and number word to numerosity representations. The prefrontal cortex is responsible for learning new facts and procedures. The parietal lobe is involved in simple and complex calculations. Multiple studies have demonstrated reduced activation of the parietal lobe in youth with MLDs relative to their peers when participating in numerosity tasks, reduced gray matter in the parietal lobe (ie, intraparietal sulcus) in individuals with MLDs, and differences in connectivity within the parietal regions and between the parietal and occipitotemporal regions. Given this pattern of deficits in key areas related to learning math and between brain regions associated with learning math, there has been a growing recognition that differential deficits in and between these brain regions may partly explain the heterogeneity in the presentation of MLD in youth.

Collectively there is growing recognition that these neurobiological differences between youth with and without reading disorder and/or MLD may offer insights into more effectively treating these disorders. For instance, some interventions that have focused on MLD have attempted to directly target the numerosity system in the intraparietal sulcus.[79] Interventions for reading disorder have found benefits in improving patterns of neural functioning associated with reading,[80] thereby allowing for more refined understanding of how these interventions improve outcomes that will, ultimately, allow for more personalized decision making regarding which treatments should be used for which individuals, based on baseline neuromarkers of treatment response. The future seems ripe for further investigation in these areas, as advances in technology allow for more precise measurement and development of personalized approaches to treatment. At present, however, despite the enthusiasm for the potential that may exist for such approaches, these interventions and methods are not ready for "prime-time"; clinicians must consider how best to target various neurobiological deficits with existing treatments and approaches.

REFERENCES

1. Shaywitz SE, Gruen JR, Shaywitz BA. Management of dyslexia, its rationale, and underlying neurobiology. Pediatr Clin North Am 2007;54(3):609–23, viii.
2. National Institute of Child Health and Human Development. Report of the National Reading Panel. Teaching children to read: An evidence-based assessment of the scientific research literature on reading and its implications for reading instruction (NIH Publication No. 00-4769). Washington, DC: U.S. Government Printing Office; 2000.
3. Handler SM, Fierson WM, Section on Ophthalmology. Learning disabilities, dyslexia, and vision. Pediatrics 2011;127(3):e818–56.
4. Shaywitz SE, Shaywitz BA. The science of reading and dyslexia. J AAPOS 2003; 7(3):158–66.
5. Alexander AW, Slinger-Constant AM. Current status of treatments for dyslexia: critical review. J Child Neurol 2004;19(10):744–58.
6. Lindamood C, Lindamood P. Phoneme sequencing program (LIPS). Austin (TX): PRO-ED; 1998.
7. Corporation SL. Fast ForWord companion: a comprehensive guide to the training exercises. Berkeley (CA): Author; 1999.
8. Saenz L, Fuchs L, Fuchs D. Peer-assisted learning strategies for English language learners with learning disabilities. Except Child 2005;71(3):231–47.
9. Torgesen J, Rashotte C, Alexander A. Progress towards understanding the instructional conditions necessary for remediating reading difficulties in older children. In: Foorman BR, editor. Preventing and remediating reading difficulties: bringing science to scale. Timonium (MD): York Press; 2003. p. 275–98.
10. Lovett MW, Lea L, Borden SL, et al. Components of effective remediation for developmental reading disabilities: combining phonological and strategy-based instruction to improve outcomes. J Educ Psychol 2000;92(2):263–83.
11. Oakland T, Black JL, Stanford G, et al. An evaluation of the dyslexia training program: a multisensory method for promoting reading in students with reading disabilities. J Learn Disabil 1998;31(2):140–7.
12. Hook P, Jones S, Macaruzo P. The efficacy of FastForWord training on facilitating acquisition of reading skills in children with specific reading disabilities—a longitudinal study. Ann Dyslexia 2001;51:75–96.
13. Torgesen J, Wagner R, Rashotte C, et al. Preventing reading failure in young children with phonological processing disabilities: group and individual responses to instruction. J Educ Psychol 1999;91(4):579–93.
14. Torgesen J, Alexander A, Wagner R, et al. Intensive remedial instruction for children with severe reading disabilities: immediate and long-term outcomes from two instructional approaches. J Learn Disabil 2001;34(1):33–58, 78.
15. Pokorni J, Worthington C, Jamison P. Phonological awareness intervention: comparison of Fast ForWord, Earobics, and LiPS. J Educ Res 2004;97:147–57.
16. Temple E, Deutsch GK, Poldrack RA, et al. Neural deficits in children with dyslexia ameliorated by behavioral remediation: evidence from functional MRI. Proc Natl Acad Sci U S A 2003;100(5):2860–5.
17. Fuchs L, Fuchs D, Phillips N, et al. Acquisition and transfer effects of classwide peer-assisted learning strategies in mathematics for students with varying learning histories. Sch Psychol Rev 1995;24(4):604–20.

18. Fuchs D, Fuchs L, Mathes P, et al. Peer-assisted learning strategies: making classrooms more responsive to diversity. Am Educ Res J 1997;34(1):174–206.

19. Duffy G, Roehler L, Meloth M, et al. The relationship between explicit verbal explanations during reading skill instruction and students' awareness and achievement: a study of reading teacher effects. Read Res Q 1986;21:237–50.

20. Rosenshine B. Explicit teaching. In: Berliner DC, Rosenshine BV, editors. Talks to teachers: a festschrift for N. L. Gage. New York: Random House; 1987. p. 75–92.

21. What Works Clearinghouse. What Works Clearinghouse intervention report. Institute of Education Sciences; 2012. http://www.ies.ed.gov/ncee/wwc/pdf/intervention_reports/wwc_pals_060512.pdf. Accessed September 15, 2012.

22. American Academy of Pediatrics, Section on Ophthalmology, Council on Children with Disabilities, et al. Joint statement–learning disabilities, dyslexia, and vision. Pediatrics 2009;124(2):837–44.

23. Maccini P, Mulcahy CA, Wilson MG. A follow-up of mathematics interventions for secondary students with learning disabilities. Learn Disabil Res Pract 2007; 22(1):58–74.

24. Geary CD. Mathematics and learning disabilities. J Learn Disabil 2004;37(1):4.

25. Powell SR, Fuchs LS, Fuchs D, et al. Effects of fact retrieval tutoring on third-grade students with math difficulties with and without reading difficulties. Learn Disabil Res Pract 2009;24(1):1–11.

26. Hasselbring TS, Goin LJ, Bransford JD. Developing math automaticity in learning handicapped children: the role of computerized drill and practice. Focus Except Child 1988;20(6):1–7.

27. Okolo CM. The effect of computer-assisted instruction format and initial attitude on the arithmetic facts proficiency and continuing motivation of students with learning disabilities. Exceptionality 1992;3(4):195–211.

28. Fuchs LS, Fuchs D, Hamlet CL, et al. The Effects of computer-assisted instruction on number combination skill in at-risk first graders. J Learn Disabil 2006; 39(5):467.

29. Witzel BS. Using CRA to teach algebra to students with math difficulties in inclusive settings. Learn Disabil 2005;3(2):49–60.

30. Maccini P, Hughes CA. Effects of a problem-solving strategy on the introductory algebra performance of secondary. Learn Disabil Res Pract 2000;15(1):10.

31. Butler FM, Miller SP, Crehan K, et al. Fraction instruction for students with mathematics disabilities: comparing two teaching sequences. Learn Disabil Res Pract 2003;18(2):99.

32. Witzel BS, Mercer CD, Miller DM. Teaching algebra to students with learning difficulties: an investigation of an explicit instruction model. Learn Disabil Res Pract 2003;18(2):121.

33. Montague M, Enders C, Dietz S. Effects of cognitive strategy instruction on math problem solving of middle school students with learning disabilities. Learn Disabil Q 2011;34(4):262.

34. Montague M. Cognitive strategy instruction in mathematics for students with learning disabilities. J Learn Disabil 1997;30(2):164.

35. Test DW, Ellis MF. The effects of LAP fractions on addition and subtraction of fractions with students with mild disabilities. Educ Treat Children 2005;28(1): 11–24.

36. Manalo E, Bunnell JK, Stillman JA. The use of process mnemonics in teaching students with mathematics learning disabilities. Learn Disabil Q 2000;23(2):137.

37. Jitendra A, DiPipi CM, Perron-Jones N. An exploratory study of schema-based word-problem–solving instruction for middle school students with learning

disabilities: an emphasis on conceptual and procedural understanding. J Spec Educ 2002;36(1):23–38.

38. Jitendra AK, Hoff K, Beck MM. Teaching middle school students with learning disabilities to solve word problems using a schema-based approach. Remedial Special Education 1999;20(1):50.

39. Xin YP, Jitendra AK, Deatline-Buchman A. Effects of mathematical word problem-solving instruction on middle school students with learning problems. J Spec Educ 2005;39(3):181–92.

40. Graham S, Harris KR. Evidence-based writing practices: drawing recommendations from multiple sources. Br J Educ Psychol 2009;1:95–111.

41. Rogers LA, Graaham S. A meta-analysis of single-subject design writing intervention research. J Educ Psychol 2008;100:879–906.

42. Graham S, Harris KR. Students with learning disabilities and the process of writing. A meta-analysis of SRSD studies. In: Harris KR, Graham S, editors. Handbook of research on learning disabilities. New York: Guilford Press; 2003. p. 383–402.

43. Taft R, Mason L. Examining effects of writing interventions: highlighting results for students with primary disabilities other than learning disabilities. Remedial Special Education 2001;32:359–70.

44. Rabipour S, Raz A. Training the brain: fact and fad in cognitive and behavioral remediation. Brain Cogn 2012;79(2):159–79.

45. Holmes J, Gathercole SE, Dunning DL. Adaptive training leads to sustained enhancement of poor working memory in children. Dev Sci 2009;12(4):F9–15.

46. Klingberg T, Fernell E, Olesen PJ, et al. Computerized training of working memory in children with ADHD—a randomized, controlled trial. J Am Acad Child Adolesc Psychiatry 2005;44(2):177–86.

47. Olesen PJ, Westerberg H, Klingberg T. Increased prefrontal and parietal activity after training of working memory. Nat Neurosci 2004;7(1):75–9.

48. Brehmer Y, Westerberg H, Backman L. Working-memory training in younger and older adults: training gains, transfer, and maintenance. Front Hum Neurosci 2012;6:63.

49. Green CT, Long DL, Green D, et al. Will working memory training generalize to improve off-task behavior in children with attention-deficit/hyperactivity disorder? Neurotherapeutics 2012;9(3):639–48.

50. Shipstead Z, Redick TS, Engle EC. CogMed working memory training: does the evidence support the claims? J Appl Res Mem Cogn 2012;1:185–93.

51. Shipstead Z, Redick TS, Engle RW. Is working memory training effective? Psychol Bull 2012;138(4):628–54.

52. Hulme C, Melby-Lervag M. Current evidence does not support the claims made for Cogmed working memory training. J Appl Res Mem Cogn 2012;1:197–200.

53. Morrison A, Chein J. The controversy of Cogmed. J Appl Res Mem Cogn 2012; 1:208–10.

54. Melby-Lervag M, Hulme C. Is working memory training effective? A meta-analytic review. Dev Psychol 2012;49(2):270–91.

55. Klingberg T, Forssberg H, Westerberg H. Training of working memory in children with ADHD. J Clin Exp Neuropsychol 2002;24(6):781–91.

56. Beck SJ, Hanson CA, Puffenberger SS, et al. A controlled trial of working memory training for children and adolescents with ADHD. J Clin Child Adolesc Psychol 2010;39(6):825–36.

57. American Speech-Language Hearing Association. (Central) auditory processing disorders [Technical report]. 2005.

58. Fey ME, Richard GJ, Geffner D, et al. Auditory processing disorder and auditory/language interventions: an evidence-based systematic review. Lang Speech Hear Serv Sch 2011;42(3):246–64.
59. Yencer KA. Clinical focus: grand rounder. The effects of auditory integration training for children with central auditory processing disorders. Am J Audiol 1998;7(2):32–44.
60. Gilmor T. The efficacy of the Tomatis method for children with learning and communication disorders: a meta analysis. International Journal of Listening 1999;13:12–23.
61. Ross-Swain D. The effects of auditory stimulation on auditory processing disorder: a summary of the findings. International Journal of Listening 2007;21:140–55.
62. Hayes EA, Warrier CM, Nicol TG, et al. Neural plasticity following auditory training in children with learning problems. Clin Neurophysiol 2003;114(4):673–84.
63. Russo NM, Nicol TG, Zecker SG, et al. Auditory training improves neural timing in the human brainstem. Behav Brain Res 2005;156(1):95–103.
64. Warrier CM, Johnson KL, Hayes EA, et al. Learning impaired children exhibit timing deficits and training-related improvements in auditory cortical responses to speech in noise. Exp Brain Res 2004;157(4):431–41.
65. Miller CA, Uhring EA, Brown JJ, et al. Case studies of auditory training for children with auditory processing difficulties: a preliminary analysis. Contemp Issues Commun Sci Disord 2005;32:93–107.
66. Deppeler JM, Taranto AM, Bench J. Language and auditory processing changes following Fast ForWord. Aust New Zeal J Audiol 2004;26(2):94–109.
67. Merzenich MM, Jenkins WM, Johnston P, et al. Temporal processing deficits of language-learning impaired children ameliorated by training. Science 1996;271(5245):77–81.
68. Stevens C, Fanning J, Coch D, et al. Neural mechanisms of selective auditory attention are enhanced by computerized training: electrophysiological evidence from language-impaired and typically developing children. Brain Res 2008;1205:55–69.
69. Tallal P, Miller SL, Bedi G, et al. Language comprehension in language-learning impaired children improved with acoustically modified speech. Science 1996;271(5245):81–4.
70. Cohen W, Hodson A, O'Hare A, et al. Effects of computer-based intervention through acoustically modified speech (Fast ForWord) in severe mixed receptive-expressive language impairment: outcomes from a randomized controlled trial. J Speech Lang Hear Res 2005;48(3):715–29.
71. Gillam R, Loeb D, Hoffman L, et al. The efficacy of Fast ForWord Language intervention in school-age children with language impairment: a randomized controlled trial. J Speech Lang Hear Res 2008;51(1):97–119.
72. Nelson JR, Benner GJ, Gonzalez J. Learner characteristics that influence the treatment effectiveness of early literacy interventions: a meta-analytic review. Learn Disabil Res Pract 2003;18:255–67.
73. Frijters J, Lovett M, Steinback K, et al. Neurocognitive predictors of reading outcomes for children with reading disabilities. J Learn Disabil 2011;44(2):150–66.
74. Cutting LE, Clements-Stephens A, Pugh KR, et al. Not all reading disabilities are dyslexia: distinct neurobiology of specific comprehension deficits. Brain Connect 2012. http://dx.doi:10.1089/brain.2012.0116. [Epub ahead of print].
75. Mabbott D, Bisanz J. Computational skills, working memory, and conceptual knowledge in older children with mathematics learning disabilities. J Learn Disabil 2008;41(1):15–28.

76. Gibson BS, Kronenberger WG, Gondoli DM, et al. Component analysis of simple span vs. complex span adaptive working memory exercises: a randomized, controlled trial. J Appl Res Mem Cogn 2012;1:179–84.
77. Peterson RL, Pennington BF. Developmental dyslexia. Lancet 2012;26: 1997–2007.
78. Butterworth B, Varma S, Laurillard D. Dyscalculia: from brain to education. Science 2011;332:1049–53.
79. Wilson A, Revkin SK, Cohen D, et al. An open trial assessment of "the Number Race", an adaptive computer game for remediation of dyscalculia. Behav Brain Funct 2006;2(1):2–20.
80. Gabrieli JD. Dyslexia: a new synergy between education and cognitive neuro-science. Science 2009;17:280–3.

Paradigm Shift: Stages of Physicians' Entry into Integrative Practice

Scott Shannon, MD, ABIHM[a,b],*

KEYWORDS

- Integrative medicine • Philosophic paradigm • Integrative mental health
- Stages of practice • Clinic design • Collaboration • Professional development

KEY POINTS

- The division between conventional allopathic ("against disease") medicine and integrative medicine stands clearer and more rooted in a distinct philosophic divide between rationalists and empiricists.
- Rationalists prioritize efficacy and are more driven by the power of treatments to fight the disease. Empiricists focus on the observable effects of various different treatments or actions on health.
- The two paradigms reflect reductionism and holism. Neither is right or wrong.
- Integrative medicine represents the extension of holistic medicine as it enters academic medicine.
- The learning curve in integrative medicine is huge and is only limited by the scope of one's intellectual curiosity and ambition.

INTRODUCTION

Much like the overarching framework of a child's life, the process of learning, practicing, and incorporating integrative child psychiatry can be viewed as a developmental trajectory. As we consider this process, it is useful to break it down into a few distinct steps. Any classification system is arbitrary and artificial. However, it becomes useful for consideration and discussion of this process. The organization of this article reflects this progression:

1. Paradigms
2. Doubt
3. Consideration

Disclosures: Dr Shannon has written or edited 2 prior books in this field.
[a] Department of Psychiatry, University of Colorado, Anschutz Medical Campus, Building 500, Mail Stop F546, 13001 East 17th Place, Aurora, CO 80045, USA; [b] Wholeness Center, 2620 East Prospect Road, Suite #190, Fort Collins, CO 80525, USA
* Wholeness Center, 2620 East Prospect Road, Suite #190, Fort Collins, CO 80525.
E-mail address: scott@wholeness.com

Child Adolesc Psychiatric Clin N Am 22 (2013) 479–491
http://dx.doi.org/10.1016/j.chc.2013.03.004
1056-4993/13/$ – see front matter © 2013 Elsevier Inc. All rights reserved.

PARADIGMS

The practice of child and adolescent psychiatry represents an enormous and challenging task. The complexities of the human brain overwhelm our ability to grasp it, much less the myriad complications that arise from it. It should come as no surprise that there are many different styles and approaches to how to evaluate and care for young people with mental health issues. Our practice style tends to be based on our underlying philosophy. Do we emphasize family dynamics or neurotransmitters, or psychodynamic conflicts as the explanation of our behavior? The current state of affairs in modern psychiatry precludes most of us from arriving at a simple, single philosophic orientation. Most of us see a kernel of truth in each realm that we explore, and this pulls us to the more pragmatic but confusing "eclectic" perspective that embraces all and precludes none. For many, this multifaceted philosophic complexity leaves us at times feeling disoriented with no clear pole star to navigate by. For others, the multidimensional concepts and treatments are aides that promote more effective treatment and facilitate developmental change.

One clear philosophic divide does exist. The division between conventional allopathic ("against disease") medicine and integrative medicine stands clearer and more rooted in a distinct philosophic divide, which has been present for thousands of years in medicine, going back to the Hippocratic era. Physicians since then can be divided into two distinct camps driven by a fundamental paradigmatic choice.

1. Empiricists are practitioners who believe in the healing power of the body and prefer safe, natural treatments to foster health.
2. Rationalists, on the other hand, believe that disease is a battle to be fought using rational principles to guide the attack.

Rationalists prioritize efficacy and are more driven by the power of treatments to fight the disease. Empiricists focus on the observable effects of various different treatments or actions on health, whereas rationalists tend to focus on mechanisms and scientific explanations to formulate their treatments. Conventional medicine conceptualizes primarily in terms of biochemistry and physiology (serotonin, limbic system), whereas holistic medicine thinks in terms of the integrated whole person (diet, spirituality). Perhaps more than rationalists, empiricists are more driven by the risk of harm to the body's innate healing power, and thus prioritize safety. Empiricists tend to prefer gentler treatments and are typically more comfortable with taking considerable time for healing. Rationalists often prefer a more aggressive style of treatment, and seem to have less patience for slow response. Early holistic physicians adopted healing treatments from all over the globe, especially traditional medical systems that have stood the test of time, whereas conventional physicians focused on randomized controlled trials and tended to value methods developed in more economically advanced countries.

In modern health care, the rise of evidence-based medicine (EBM) has brought the value of scientifically demonstrated efficacy to the forefront as never before. We have a multitude of grading scales that categorize the existing individual research studies in terms of the efficacy of the examined treatments. Safety concerns have also driven some similar scales, but these have penetrated clinical practice to a lesser degree. Most practitioners would agree that finding an effective and safe treatment stands as a universal goal in the care of an individual patient. However, there are few treatments that are both completely effective and totally safe. Ultimately, each practitioner must select one of these two goals as the priority in treatment selection for each individual patient. In the clinical arena we must choose between actual treatments that differ widely in terms of documented efficacy and safety. There is no ideal treatment: one must select based on some priority. For modern conventional medicine it is effectiveness that drives decision making, whereas holistic practitioners place the priority on safety. This dichotomy reflects the deep and persisting divide between two health care paradigms (Shannon, Weil, and Kaplan, 2011).

The paradigmatic divide can be observed in the United States over the last 200 years. During the cholera epidemics that swept through the United States in the 1830s, the allopaths used bloodletting, purging with calomel (mercury salts), and emetics to rid the body of the toxic invasion. The homeopaths used safe homeopathic remedies to strengthen the body. Not surprisingly, the homeopaths fared better and gained in popularity. It is unclear whether the allopaths created more iatrogenic deaths or that homeopathy was an effective treatment, or both. We may never know. The American Medical Association was formed in 1847 to counter the resultant rise of homeopathy in the United States. The homeopaths and others from the Empiricist camp (naturopaths, osteopaths, herbalists, and so forth) have continued to exist in American health over the ensuing decades.

The Flexner Report of 1910 purged Empiricists from the ranks of allopathic medicine by narrowing training and practice. At that time, homeopathic hospitals and medical schools were common in the United States. In the 1960s and 1970s, the empiric approach reappeared in the form of physicians embracing a perspective of prevention, nutrition, and natural treatments that ran counter to the prevailing allopathic doctrine.

The two paradigms reflect reductionism and holism. Neither is right or wrong. Our brain has two hemispheres: the left is reductionistic and the right is holistic. These ways of looking at the world and evaluating information are both valid. Reductionism offers detailed knowledge and more specific information. Holism offers wisdom and context. We need both in order to function well in the world and practice medicine. Our society tends to move back and forth between extremes of these two different modes. Rationalism reflects reductionist thought, and Empiricism models more holism. Obtaining balance between the two may be the most important goal for a physician. Some would argue that modern conventional medicine has moved to such a reductionistic extreme that holism becomes ever more attractive as a path to find greater balance.

Perhaps complementary and alternative medicine (CAM) and holistic medicine offer certain benefits that many crave: more personalized attention, greater wisdom about lifestyle, and a unity of body, mind, and spirit. Thus, this paradigm shift toward holism may be part of a broader healing process for society. Many, myself (the author, S.S.) included, think of medicine as an applied social science that is driven in various ways by societal factors outside of what we traditionally think of as science. In an ecosystems model, health functions on many levels. One of the underlying tenets of holistic medicine is that a life force within us pulls us to higher levels of order and balance all the time. I would speculate that once societies move to extremes, factors emerge that begin to seek a healing balance as a homeostatic process.

The undercurrent originally called holistic medicine has continued to grow and expand. It was renamed integrative medicine in the mid-1990s, a term popularized by Andrew Weil, who established the first Fellowship in Integrative Medicine at the University of Arizona in 1997. This practice style has continued to spread and grow. At present, the Consortium of Academic Health Centers in Integrative Medicine counts 51 medical schools in the United States as members. CAM is the term most broadly used by the public. What is the philosophic process underlying this rapid growth of CAM in the United States?

Each field of science creates a specific paradigm or belief system, or set of systems, to understand a broad field of inquiry. Medicine is but one scientific paradigm. Scientific paradigms as outlined by Thomas Kuhn (1962) go through their own process of growth and change. At times, one scientific paradigm will reach a point at which it will rapidly give way to another competing perspective. Many different external processes can accelerate this paradigm shift. In the case of integrative medicine, the popular demand for natural and holistic care has been one trigger speeding or driving this process, which has appeared to be a grass-roots shift from one paradigm (conventional/rationalist) to another (holistic/empiricist). The momentum for this current paradigm shift in medicine has been accelerated by strong consumer demand and public interest. More recently, we have witnessed increasing curiosity about the holistic paradigm by a younger generation of physicians. The demographics for integrative medicine show particularly strong interest with the young, well educated, and affluent, who are often the leaders of societal change.

In medicine today, we have two distinct paradigms for practice:

1. Conventional allopathic care
2. CAM-oriented holistic care

Integrative medicine represents the extension of holistic medicine as it enters academic medicine. Most of this article is devoted to exploring the process as a physician moves from the current dominant perspective in conventional care to what is still a minority perspective, in a shift of underlying philosophic paradigms. For the general public, CAM has already achieved a kind of dominance, as there are more visits to CAM providers each year than to primary care physicians. This transformation does not reflect a uniform process for all practitioners, but enough commonalities emerge to make this discussion valuable, particularly for physicians moving through it. The goal of this article is to consider this process and to support providers immersed in this process.

DOUBT

As practicing child and adolescent psychiatrists, we can be caught in the paradigm shift ourselves. The vast majority of us were primarily schooled in conventional thought and practice through our medical training and psychiatric residency. In the past, and to a significant degree still now, the attitudes toward CAM in most conventional training programs range from complete ignorance to frank hostility. Even today, the typical psychiatrist encounters very little exposure to any CAM in residency unless they seek it out. Thus, most new psychiatrists still embrace the conventional allopathic paradigm by default, even though they may be less philosophically hostile to CAM than prior generations of psychiatrists. As practitioners, their treatments remain predominantly guided by allopathic limitations.

We move through our training and launch into the practice of our chosen profession. Soon, the harsh realities of managing and treating patients becomes obvious: Our diagnostic system is not always clear, our medications do not always work, many patients encounter significant side effects, our psychotherapies receive scant support from managed care, patients and families often express interest in treatment options that you know little about (like CAM), your satisfaction level suffers from being relegated to mainly writing prescriptions, but, most of all, you do not see the progress in your patients that you once envisioned. Practice seems all too often frustrating, boring, limited, or draining.

Perhaps most of all, you begin to doubt your tools. Some nonconventional treatments begin to appeal to you. Your doubt and dissatisfaction grows. You ask yourself: "Did I make the right career choice?" Another large group of providers move through a different journey. You look with curiosity at other styles of practice, other types of research, and even other treatment philosophies. This path offers some new options, perhaps additional tools for our basket of professional skills. Curiosity and the relentless search for knowledge is a drive to action.

Resources:
    Capra F. The web of life. New York: Anchor Books; 1997.
    Kuhn T. The structure of scientific revolutions. Chicago: University of Chicago Press; 1962.
    Shannon S, Weil A, Kaplan B. Medical decision making in integrative medicine. Alternative Compl Ther 2011;17(2):84–91.

CONSIDERATION

From this place of doubt, you begin to explore other options. Surely, there has to be more. What about all of these supplements your patients ask about? What is going on in all those health food stores? You notice flyers for professional training in herbal medicine, acupuncture, or functional medicine. What is this stuff? You feel overwhelmed or avoidant, as it is foreign territory and completely novel to you. Yet something about it intrigues you, perhaps grabs you on an emotional or intuitive level. Or perhaps you have seen it work for friends, even though it does not fit your scientific model or mechanistic understanding.

As you move fully into the consideration phase, you begin to read articles, explore the Internet, perhaps buy books, ask friends and colleagues about it. At some point, you may begin to think about and even explore the science behind it. The field is relatively new to modern medicine, the research base is emerging, yet something makes sense to you: the caution about risk, the focus on diet/nutrition, the healing power of the body, the integration of body-mind-spirit, the centuries of traditional practice, and the power of the mind. So you begin to explore how to incorporate some new elements into your practice. You begin to dabble.

Resources:
    Weil A. Health and healing. New York: Mariner Books; 2004.
    Weil A. Spontaneous healing. New York: Ballantine Books; 2000.

DABBLING

The next phase involves the cautious application of a few novel treatment options. Maybe it is fish oil or SAM-e (S-adenosyl methionine). You have to sort out how to use it and where to get it. To some, part of this process seems illicit, undercover, almost like it is illegal. What would your teachers have said? What will the administrators think? You may have some fears about your legal liability. What is my risk if I use vitamins instead of prescription agents? Can I be sued if I discuss nutrition or recommend acupuncture, especially if it fails? What will my partners or colleagues think of me? Will the therapists in town stop referring? What if my information about the treatment is wrong? You might make some tentative inquiries to your board of medical examiners or insurance carriers about this topic as you feel some real caution.

Gradually, cautiously, hesitantly, you try on some "outside the box" approaches in your own practice. Some patients get better (and some do not). You notice that parents appreciate the extra options you offer. You feel encouraged by the successes, grow a bit bolder, and expand the options. You read about additional treatments. Something about these tools seems a bit more congruent to you.

Suddenly, at some point, you realize that you feel like you are straddling two worlds. You have one foot in the conventional model that you trained in and one foot in the world of CAM. You feel the split, the tension between these two world views. Some will be comfortable with a conventionally based practice augmented with a few CAM options and keep an open mind. Others feel drawn to go further.

Resources:
Lake J. Textbook of integrative mental health. New York: Thieme; 2009.
Lake J, Spiegel D. Complementary and alternative treatments in mental health. Arlington (VA): American Psychiatric Publishing; 2007.
Shannon S. Handbook of complementary and alternative treatments in mental health. San Diego (CA): Academic Press; 2002.

PERSONAL CONVERSION

A big step occurs when your own self-care begins to change. When you reach for Echinacea instead of Nyquil. When you change your diet instead of using Nexium. When you decide to practice yoga instead of taking Ambien. When acupuncture makes more sense to you than an epidural injection of steroids. At this point, your world view has begun to shift; you are transitioning from the more reductionistic model of allopathic medicine to the more holistic model of CAM. From epigenetics to neuroplasticity to ecology, modern science increasingly endorses the interactive systems perspective of holism. It mirrors the movement of physics from the perspective of Newton to the relativity of Einstein.

At some point in this process, you may cross a threshold, bringing both feet into the perspective of integrative medicine. There is a point of no return. Once your mindset, your world view, and your health care paradigm shifts to include CAM perspectives and treatments, it is impossible to see patients or your practice the same way again. You have reached the point of personal conversion. You now embrace more than CAM tools, you embrace the paradigm of holism. You think about health, healing, and the powers of the body, and you function as a healer quite differently. Now you are hungry to learn how to work in a different manner.

For some, this process is less uniform and more segmented. The growing acceptance of holistic principles and treatments may come bit by bit. Practice change may lead philosophic conversion, or vice versa. Personality factors also play a significant role here as well. In the early years of holistic medicine, it was a frontier community of iconoclasts, renegades, and pioneers. People of firm conviction and strong opinions were not afraid to step out of the box and into the fire. Practitioners with hesitation, doubt, or caution need not have applied. Now, as we move into the "early adopter" phase, the process of conversion includes a much wider range of styles and personalities. In turn, the process itself tends to less consistent and often less dramatic.

Resources:

Kemper K. Mental health naturally. Elk Grove Village (IL): American Academy of Pediatrics; 2010.

Shannon S. Mental health for the whole child. New York: Norton; 2013.

Shannon S. Please don't label my child. New York: Rodale; 2007.

TRAINING

At this stage in your hunger for tools and techniques, you jump into your new-found passion. You start to read voraciously and attend a wide variety of seminars, workshops, and conferences. For most practitioners, even living in large urban centers, this may involve some travel. You may consider retraining in an integrative medicine residency program, but retooling may be financially or pragmatically unfeasible. But you may feel a sense of conflict or even incompleteness about your level of medical expertise. You may begin to feel that you are not the full clinician that you had always hoped to view yourself as being. Nonetheless, your interest and passion drives you, and you find ways to expand your involvement and commitment. You might settle for a detailed reading of an integrative medicine textbook or subscribe to some CAM journals.

As a psychiatrist, as you see the way that the psychiatrically targeted CAM treatments operate and interact with a variety of physiologic systems apart from the central nervous system, you realize that you need to become much more comfortable with a much broader range of knowledge in health care. The gut, the thyroid, the adrenals, diet, inflammation, detoxification, and many other disparate arenas become critical topics to consider for understanding your patient. All of a sudden, biochemistry topics like methylation and folate metabolism rise from slumber in the deep recesses of your memory and become essential to understanding the treatments you are using. Perhaps acupuncture, homeopathy, Ayurveda, or herbal medicine draws some interest, but the scope of data can overwhelm with the burden of new learning. Even vitamins and minerals may seem like too large an area to master. But you are a physician, you are accustomed to studying hard, and you push yourself ahead: It is amazing what a rekindled passion for medicine and psychiatry can foster. You feel an enthusiasm that you have not felt since the days of your residency.

Resources:

Rakel D. Textbook of integrative medicine. New York: Elsevier; 2012. This is the classic textbook for integrative medicine.

American Board of Integrative Holistic Medicine: www.abihm.org. This organization offers a week-long comprehensive board review course and a certifying examination for physicians, which is an excellent means to obtain a broad overview of the science and practice of this emerging field. This course reconnects psychiatrists with the other arenas of health care. More than 1700 physicians have been certified, and this network and Web site are helpful for finding appropriate physicians for patient referrals.

Consortium of Academic Health Centers in Integrative Medicine: www.imconsortium.org. This group represents more than 50 academic health centers in the United States. The Consortium is an excellent resource for patient referrals, consultation, and inspiration for what integrative care can look like. The Consortium now offers 11 fellowship programs for training in integrative medicine.

PRACTICE

Through your dabbling, you have found a range of acceptance and skepticism from colleagues or administrators, but your patients have been very enthusiastic about the options you bring to them. You start to see real healing and recovery in some patients, and not just maintenance. As you invest increasing amounts of time and energy into mastering new realms of knowledge, you begin to reconsider the bigger picture about the way that you practice medicine. You start to dream about new styles of practice. Perhaps some elements of your current work begin to assume a bit of a negative emotional tone for you. You talk to others about different ways to see patients and to set up practice. You feel restlessness within that seems foreign. There are now parts of your old style of practice that just do not feel right or even reasonable any more. You begin to think about making deeper changes.

At this point, your practice begins to shift and change. Perhaps you develop new interests and focus on different clinical issues. You see treatment and healing from a different perspective. You realize the vast array of healing options that exist. As you look at things more holistically, you begin to ponder on how your skill set, valuable as it is, reflects just a part of what your patients need for healing. You begin to look beyond yourself to other practitioners who have altered their practices.

Resources:

Institute for Functional Medicine: www.functionalmedicine.org. This organization represents a rapidly growing segment of CAM that focuses on metabolic testing, gut health, nutrition, inflammation and detoxification. The Institute offers a wide range of training modules that are well delivered.

Center for Mind-Body Medicine: www.cmbm.org. Started by James Gordon, a pioneering psychiatrist, this organization trains health care professionals in mind-body medicine and nutrition. The course, called Food as Medicine, is a solid cornerstone for anyone interested in integrative medicine.

Helms Medical Institute: www.hmieducation.com. For more than 30 years, Joe Helms has organized the premier course in medical acupuncture in the United States. Dr Helms has trained the vast majority of physicians who practice medical acupuncture in the United States. His course is well run and is geared toward practicing physicians.

University of Arizona Program in Integrative Medicine. The University of Arizona, my alma mater, has become the single largest training program in integrative medicine. Set up as a distance learning program, the fellowship covers 2 years and trains more than 100 physicians per year.

COLLABORATION

One of the major draws for practitioners in the holistic paradigm is the opportunity to work with others and function as a team. Working as a team embodies the notion of holism and downplays our wish to believe that we can "do it all." One of the major hindrances of modern conventional care is the "silo" fragmentation that makes the patient (and often the practitioner) feel like a cog in an impersonal machine. The benefits of collaboration draw people together. This process can occur in several different ways.

In the solo collaboration model, you work in collaboration with other individual integrative practitioners in your community or region. In effect, you set up a functional clinic without walls. You identify a group of skilled practitioners in your local community or region that can work well with you to provide comprehensive integrative care across medical specialties. In the solo collaboration model, you evaluate and treat patients from your psychiatric perspective and refer out for other CAM mental health and general medical services that you do not provide. All of you work together as a team. You provide services as an integrative or holistic psychiatrist.

By being known in your community as a psychiatrist who provides CAM treatments, you have stepped out on our own and have come out of the closet. You call yourself an integrative psychiatrist. Based on prior CAM treatments that you have offered, or consultations to conventional psychiatrists in which you explain some CAM treatments, many in your community may already identify you as a CAM or integrative psychiatrist. As you step into that role, you have a few major decisions to make.

There are some practical issues that arise along the way. Will you accept insurance? This is a major question. You find that insurance reimburses you for time with an individual patient, but it does not cover supplements, certain testing, or most other CAM services. Insurance pushes us toward a higher volume and a lower reimbursement model that many find frustrating; not to mention the paperwork, denials, prior authorizations, and so forth. Do you go to a cash model? A cash model may not work in certain practices, such as with more indigent populations. Many struggle with the elitist feel of a cash practice. The cash option seems more attractive but limits your clientele to some degree. Insurance limits you in some ways, but seems more predictable.

You have some decisions to make. Will you sell dietary supplements in your office (if your state allows that)? How do you market yourself to your local referral base? Should you consider marketing to patients more directly? What do you tell your malpractice carrier? These considerations vary by person and circumstance, and sound guidance is critical.

As you explore the feasibility of a more collaborative practice, it is helpful to talk with key members of your referral base to discuss the new types of treatment you are offering, and to explain changes in your practice. It is also helpful to visit various CAM practitioners in your region, perhaps for lunch, and talk about how they might treat a problem from their perspective. Or you can schedule a treatment for yourself with a local CAM practitioner and experience what each practitioner does. This consultation serves many purposes. It furthers your own healing. It lets you know exactly what your colleague does and how they do it. It removes any perceived power or status differential. Ask questions, and let them teach you about their practice.

The benefits of a collaborative solo practice are the size: the care, efficiency, relative ease, and control of running your own small operation. The downsides are that collaboration is less effective and less rewarding when it is off-site. Communication is more cumbersome, and cross-disciplinary teaching is less predictable. A percentage of patients will not make the jump or will be lost in the process. You might still feel professionally isolated at times, or feel that the possibilities for more effective collaborative care are being missed.

Resources:

Business Consultants in CAM development:

Integrative Wellness Consultants: Stephen Paneblanco, MD. Dr Paneblanco works with his wife. He trained in Andrew Weil's program and offers a unique perspective on business development. www.iwaconsultants.homestead.com

SMALL CLINIC

Over time, you find the rewards of the solo collaborative model to include greater professional effectiveness, but you decide that you would like to do something more comprehensive and more ambitious. What would it take to start up your own clinic or center? The operation would become more complex, as you will involve disciplines and hire professionals that have not worked together before.

Some physicians will remain satisfied and fulfilled with a solo practice, preferring the simplicity or the sense of control. Opening a clinic is not for everyone. But in 30 years of working with CAM physicians and national organizations, I have found that most CAM physicians hold some curiosity or interest in opening a clinic: This process seems to form a common and natural extension of the movement toward a holistic perspective.

You clearly need someone with business experience to guide you. How do you share overheads and profits? Are you all owners or just you? Marketing, front office operations, and retail become much greater concerns. Do you take insurance for some or none? Do you develop a niche or try to practice more broadly? How do you create a brand?

I have seen many small clinics start up. Some do it well, some poorly. Much of this will be based on your reputation, your respect in the community, your network of referrals, your planning, and the quality of the team you select. Are they established or new to the area? Do they bring their own patients with them? Will they get out and network to market themselves and the clinic? Is there a shortage of specialists in your area or is it crowded? How are the demographics in your region? Are they friendly to CAM (young, educated, affluent)? How is your location (the West Coast, Mountain West, and Northeast are more supportive while the South and Southeast are less so)? These considerations all become critical determinants of your success.

Your own motivation and commitment to this process is also crucial. Do you have a sense of the personal and financial stress that setting up a clinic will generate? Do you have the time and energy to pull this off? How are your business skills? Could you negotiate with other practitioners? Can you deal with budgets and staff conflicts? Can you lead a group of people? The skill set for business success is quite different than that required for the practice of medicine or psychiatry. Good intentions and big heart alone will not achieve it.

A critical question for a clinic is: what people and what specialties do you invite to join you? The prime driver here is to get the right people with the ideal skill set. I see the skill set as being more flexible than getting the right people. Get to know people well before you jump in. Spend time with them. Explore some references and ask hard questions. Ask people close to you (such as your spouse) what they think about this person. In one of my early ventures, I let my enthusiasm for a project pull me into something I soon regretted because I had not vetted it with my partners sufficiently. Whether you develop a small clinic or a large one, you will be spending a lot of time with these people. Make sure they share your values and goals, but also make sure you enjoy them and like them. These persons will become family of sorts, and the chemistry will make a huge difference in how you feel about going into work each morning. I have started 5 clinics in my 30 years of medical practice, in chronologic order a holistic medical clinic, a large conventional multidisciplinary mental health group, a large multidisciplinary integrative clinic, a moderately sized hospital-based center for holistic medicine, and a large comprehensive integrative mental health clinic. The only thing that is clear to me after organizing and directing these operations is that selecting the right people far outweighs the importance of skill sets or professional discipline in creating a team that works well together.

In both the large and small clinic, an apothecary for selling dietary supplements makes sense, if it is legal in your state. Retail is a brave new world for physicians, but your patients will appreciate the convenience. It can serve as a minor profit center, but remember it does take considerable time to manage this well. You can manage this yourself, or have someone with a greater interest or background (such as a naturopath) take care of it. Obviously, the ideal skill set is also important to the success of your project.

If you are limiting your practice to child and adolescent psychiatry, the ideal mix of disciplines might look something like this:

1. Integrative child and adolescent psychiatrist with a comfort in nutrition, mind-body medicine, and/or functional medicine. Must be curious and open minded.
2. Naturopath, preferably a licensed naturopath, from 1 of the 4 accredited 4-year schools that award an ND degree. These practitioners are educated in all of the central realms of natural medicine, including nutrition, acupuncture, homeopathy, gut health, and a range of other aspects of general medicine, a broad range of CAM, and some elements of conventional treatment modalities; they are currently licensed in 16 states and 5 Canadian provinces.
3. Family therapist/individual therapist with training in a parenting program, such as the Nurtured Heart Approach, as well as expertise with individual therapy and group. Eye movement desensitization and reprocessing (EMDR) or dialectical behavior therapy (DBT) is a plus.
4. Mind-body therapist to focus on biofeedback, neurofeedback, meditation, hypnosis, and/or relaxation skills. Yoga is a plus.
5. Optional: neurofeedback (a wonderful tool for attention-deficit/hyperactivity disorder) therapist.
6. Administrator/front office: comfort with details, people, bookkeeping, billing, account management, and marketing. Billing and accounting may be farmed out.

Obviously this mix will vary by preference and availability of key people. One of each discipline is a good start. A psychologist who does testing and works with schools is another real plus.

LARGE CLINIC

The first step in setting up a large clinic is to question your thought process. Why do you want to do this? What is your goal? The challenges of planning, development, and risk increase exponentially as you increase the size of the clinic you plan to open. You have to make sure that you have the passion, tools, time, and resources to pull this off well.

You should understand that it may be 1 or 2 years (or more) until you reach a financial break-even point. You will need the finances and commitment to weather this period. It will take a lot of time and effort to open your doors, and even longer to break even. Predicting cash flow using your business plan will be a critical early process.

Planning will take many forms. Your early efforts should be directed toward team building, planning, and networking. The selection of your core team is the single biggest factor determining your success or failure. As mentioned, the creation of the core team, your clinical family of choice, stands as the primary task. The risks and rewards here are unmatched. Take your time and apply due diligence herein. Be patient for the right people to appear.

The physical setting plays a key role in planning an integrative medicine clinic. The proper look and feel can contribute to your success by enhancing the patient experience. However, I have witnessed clinic after clinic fail from the weight of excessive overheads. In the first few years, extravagant choices for decoration, furnishings, and square footage can act like an anchor pulling you under while you are building volume. The sensible arrangement would be a tight fit for space for the key practitioners, with the option to expand when patient volume warrants such a move.

Planning plays off several elements unfamiliar to many physicians, such as budgeting, payrolls, billing, and front office function. Here is where an outside business consultant can help your chances of success by being involved right from the start. Your money will be well spent in hiring additional expertise.

Any large integrative medicine mental health clinic will require significant community engagement and support to survive. Accordingly, the core team should begin building key relationships from day 1. Reach out to local schools, social services, community agencies, and parent groups. Offer to teach or consult without charge to build familiarity and goodwill. Meet routinely with therapists, primary care physicians, and key specialists. Outside therapists in particular are eager to have integrative options for their clients, and will become important advocates. This web of professionals will be a crucial factor in survival and appropriate referrals. In my experience, the better they know you, the more likely they are to identify patients who can benefit from integrative mental health care.

Networking is but one aspect of marketing. It will be very helpful to identify some brand elements early to guide you as you spread the word about your new clinic. How will you distinguish yourself from other options in mental health? What is your 30-second sound bite describing what you do? What makes you unique? Why refer to you?

Print advertising has fallen away, and the new social media options now drive modern marketing. How do you create buzz? Social media such as Facebook and Twitter can drive interest and sustain engagement for people in the 15- to 35-year age range. You will probably need to understand these media well, or get help. How do make your clinic seem relevant, important, and personal?

If you are planning a large integrative mental health clinic, it will probably need to move beyond a child/adolescent specialization and address the needs of patients of all ages. This approach broadens your market considerably and will enhance your volume. It will also color some other considerations. For example, acupuncture will make more sense, as you will encounter more pain and addiction issues. Two psychiatrists are a minimum to drive volume and service for the full age range of patients in an integrative medicine clinic:

1. Child and adolescent psychiatrist
2. Adult psychiatrist, ideally with addictions or geriatrics expertise
3. Naturopath(s) for diet, nutrition, gut, and dietary supplement expertise for the apothecary
4. Family therapist/child therapist. DBT background a must. Nurtured Heart training a plus
5. Individual therapist. For trauma work, EMDR training is a must, and Hakomi or Somatic Experiencing (body-based psychotherapies that focus on working with mindfulness and subtle somatic clues) training is a plus
6. Neurofeedback/biofeedback therapist
7. Acupuncturist, preferably with training in traditional Chinese medicine and Chinese herbs, preferably certified by the National Certification Commission for Acupuncture and Oriental Medicine (NCCAOM), the national organization that validates competency in the practice of acupuncture and oriental medicine through professional certification.
8. Massage therapy/body work/Reiki practitioner. Energy work a plus

9. Front office. These people are your face to the world; they should be warm, enthusiastic, and engaging

10. Administrator. This person can make or break your clinic. He or she needs to be a high-energy problem solver, and very attentive to details. Some experience in office management is critical.

Resources:

Andre Belanger. Mr Belanger has a wealth of experience in working with alternative medicine. He has created several large integrative clinics across the United States and Canada. www.hbbhealth.net/andre-belanger

Anicca Media. Russell Faust, MD, PhD is an integrative ENT surgeon who also runs a media-consulting group that assists physicians in marketing and branding. Dr Faust grasps the new evolution in marketing as it applies to the holistic/integrative perspective. www.AniccaMedia.com

SUMMARY

As a physician moving through this process of paradigm shift, you must sort out what you want and what setting will best serve your needs, personality, location, colleagues, and type of practice. All of your choices are very individualized and personal. Will you work alone or with 20 others? Will you set up a large integrative clinic or work in a more conventional setting? What you select must fit well for you. Also, options and choices may change over time. There is no one single practice style, location, or philosophy that is best for everyone.

Although this article sets up a continuum of steps in the evolution of a holistic practice, this does not imply that your location on the continuum is better than another, or that your location on the spectrum reflects some inner quality or depth. This continuum merely represents an arbitrary description of the complex process of a medical practitioner undergoing change and exploring a personal paradigm shift.

As you move forward into integrative medicine and integrative mental health, you will be on a constant learning curve, which is huge and only limited by the scope of your intellectual curiosity and ambition. There are many personal benefits for physicians in embracing this field: the joy of the work, the alignment of the philosophy, and our personal growth process. But the deepest joy and most profound contribution comes from the mental and physical health and the healing relationships that we establish while taking us closer to the heart of healing.

Complementary and Alternative Medicine in Child and Adolescent Psychiatry: Legal Considerations

Michael H. Cohen, JD, MBA, MFA[a], Suzanne R. Natbony, JD[a],
Ryan B. Abbott, MD, JD, MTOM[b],*

KEYWORDS

- Complementary and alternative medicine • Health law • Informed consent • Liability
- Medicolegal aspects

KEY POINTS

- All treatment decisions should be made in a child's best interests. If the child's parents make a decision, a psychiatrist may not simply override their judgment with his or her own preference, but can report the parents to state authorities or bring the case to court if the psychiatrist believes the child might be harmed by the decision.
- There is no case law regarding the use of complementary and alternative medicine (CAM) in child psychiatry, so the risk of malpractice liability in this setting is minimal. However, any deviation from customary medical practices creates an increased risk of legal liability.
- If CAM therapies are recommended, any known risks, benefits, and alternative treatments should be fully disclosed.
- As is the case with conventional medicine, physicians can reduce their personal liability by practicing good clinical medicine, obtaining informed consent, and comprehensively documenting.

COMPLEMENTARY AND ALTERNATIVE MEDICINE AND CHILD AND ADOLESCENT PSYCHIATRY

The term complementary and alternative medicine (CAM) describes a group of health care systems, practices, and products not currently considered to be part of conventional allopathic medicine.[1] Although systems of CAM (such as chiropractic, Ayurveda, homeopathy, and naturopathy) display considerable diversity, these systems share many of the same core values, such as a holistic approach to patient care and a strong emphasis on preventive medicine.[2] CAM systems and therapies may be grouped into broad categories such as natural products, mind-body medicine, and manipulative and body-based practices.[1]

The authors report no conflicts of interest.
[a] The Michael H. Cohen Law Group, 468 North Camden Drive, Beverly Hills, CA 90210, USA;
[b] Southwestern Law School, 3050 Wilshire Boulevard, Los Angeles, CA 90010, USA
* Corresponding author.
E-mail address: DrRyanAbbott@gmail.com

Child Adolesc Psychiatric Clin N Am 22 (2013) 493–507
http://dx.doi.org/10.1016/j.chc.2013.03.005
1056-4993/13/$ – see front matter © 2013 Elsevier Inc. All rights reserved.

childpsych.theclinics.com

The use of CAM in child and adolescent psychiatry is growing in the face of increasing patient demand, a growing evidence base suggesting that certain CAM therapies may be effective, and CAM's typically lower costs in comparison with the rising costs of many biomedical therapies.[3] In the United States 10% to 15% of children use some form of CAM, and these numbers are increasing.[4] However, for psychiatrists and other conventional health care providers, prescribing CAM poses both ethical and legal concerns, including:

1. How to best manage parents who insist on using a CAM therapy against medical advice
2. Whether there is a legal duty to disclose a CAM therapy as a possible treatment alternative when recommending conventional treatments
3. Whether a CAM treatment recommendation or referral to a CAM provider will expose a psychiatrist to legal liability

This article explores these concerns and provides clinical advice for promoting patient health and safety while minimizing the psychiatrist's risk. The use of integrative medicine is discussed from a legal standpoint, so clinicians should bear in mind that certain actions may not be legally required but might nonetheless be clinically advisable or even essential.

BEST-INTEREST STANDARD

It is a well-settled principle that parents have an ethical and legal obligation to make medical decisions on behalf of their minor children.[5–8] There are 2 primary reasons why parents are entrusted with this authority to consent to, or refuse, medical treatment. First, it is generally believed that children lack the knowledge, experience, and maturity to make some of life's most difficult decisions.[9] Second, parents, with the assistance of health care providers, are expected to make decisions that are in their children's best interest. Courts presume that parents know the most about their children and care for their children's well-being more than anyone else, making them the most appropriate decision makers.[5,9] Nevertheless, the law has safeguards in place to protect children from poor parental decision making; for example, all treatment decisions must be made in the child's best interest.[5,7–9]

There is no precise test to determine which treatment option serves the child's best interest. Whether the treatment option is CAM or conventional care, many factors must be weighed to determine which treatment is most appropriate, including the risks and benefits of the treatment and its alternatives, congruence of the parents' views with the child's values and beliefs, the child's psychological and emotional welfare, the family situation, and whether less intrusive treatment would be as beneficial.[6–8,10] Some of these factors may be shaped by the parents' cultural and religious backgrounds, but ultimately the decision needs to be made in the child's best interest.[11]

DISAGREEMENTS WITH PARENTS

Disagreements about the best interests of the child may arise when the parents are pushing a psychiatrist to use a specific CAM intervention, especially if the psychiatrist is not familiar with the therapy and insufficiently knowledgable about its risks or benefits; this may lead to disagreement about the best course of action. The psychiatrist has the option to take time to learn about the suggested CAM treatment and then come back to discuss the treatment with the parents. Although there is generally no legal requirement for psychiatrists to inform themselves about the parents' preferred treatment, this would be a wise approach to take clinically. It may also be a helpful negotiating stance for the psychiatrist to become familiar with the treatment, to demonstrate to parents that their preferences are being seriously considered. However, it is unlikely that a psychiatrist could be reasonably sued for rejecting a CAM treatment while refusing to become familiar with it.

If a psychiatrist and the parents cannot agree on the appropriate treatment plan for the child, the psychiatrist should fully explain his or her reasoning and answer any questions the parents may have. If the parents and the psychiatrist are still unable to come to a consensus, under normal circumstances the parents' decision should prevail, even if it is against the psychiatrist's medical preference or advice,[7,8] especially if there is medical uncertainty regarding the effects of the CAM treatment or when the risks associated with an alternative treatment are less serious,[8,12] and the clinician does not view the child as seriously endangered by the parents' decision. Of course, it may also be the case that a psychiatrist initiates the suggestion to use a CAM treatment in the face of parental objections. Here, it is even clearer that the parents' decision should prevail, given that the CAM treatment is not a widely accepted medical practice. Psychiatrists who want to use a CAM treatment should be cognizant of potential malpractice liability and professional disciplinary actions, discussed further herein.

LIMITATIONS ON PARENTS' AUTHORITY

Although parents are accorded considerable latitude in making decisions for their minor children, they are subject to limitations.[5,12] In every American jurisdiction, the state has the authority to intervene and provide necessary medical care when parental decisions seriously threaten a child's health, safety, or welfare.[5–8,13] Even religious beliefs cannot justify treatment decisions that seriously endanger a child's life or health.[12] As United States Supreme Court Justice Wiley Rutledge famously said in 1944 in *Prince v. Massachusetts,* "Parents may be free to become martyrs themselves. But it does not follow they are free, in identical circumstances, to make martyrs of their children…[14]" Courts have interpreted the *Prince* decision to require a psychiatrist to notify child welfare authorities when a psychiatrist believes the parents' decision to refuse effective treatment will cause significant harm to the child.[7,8,12] In some states, such as Massachusetts, the psychiatrist is protected from lawsuit by the parents for taking the case to court. Thus, if the physician believes that a child might be harmed by a parent's decision or inaction, the physician can take the case to court or can refer the case to the state child welfare department, which will decide whether to take the case to court. In these cases, a court will consider expert evidence about medical practices, assess the benefits and burdens of a treatment and its alternatives (including nontreatment), and determine whether to respect the parents' decision or to allow child welfare authorities to consent to the treatment.[6,15–17]

Sometimes, parents will disagree with each other over a treatment plan and may have a generally adversarial relationship. In such instances, the child's treatment can become a weapon used against the other parent. Psychiatrists should deal with this situation in the same way they handle disputes regarding conventional treatment.[18] In most states if the parents are married, either parent may consent to medical care. If married parents disagree over care, it is legally unclear whether a psychiatrist can side with one parent; in this situation, the child's preferences may come into play. If the parents are divorced or were never married, the right to consent depends on state law: The parent with legal custody may have the sole right to consent. A psychiatrist should not deny a child necessary medical care because of uncertainty, but in the case of elective care or CAM, the safest course of action is to seek a court's decision in the case.

There is limited case law regarding disagreement about CAM use between a psychiatrist and the parents. The outcomes in these cases tend to turn on expert testimony and medical evidence presented at trial, during which the recommended treatment's risks and benefits are compared with the CAM treatment's risks and benefits. This process can result in seemingly discordant legal decisions. For example, within a month of one another, two courts came to very different conclusions about whether the use of an unconventional therapy had served the child's best interest.[19] These cases involved treatment of childhood cancer with laetrile, which is not approved as a safe and effective drug under the Federal Food, Drug, and Cosmetic Act. In the first case, a New York court considered whether the parents of a 7-year-old boy with Hodgkin disease were liable for child neglect when they refused conventional care (radiation and chemotherapy) in favor of nutritional and metabolic therapies.[16] Both the parents and the state presented expert testimony on the risks and benefits of conventional care in comparison with those of laetrile.[16] The New York court ultimately concluded that because there was medical evidence supporting the use of laetrile showing that metabolic therapy had fewer risks than radiation or chemotherapy, the parents' decision to forgo the conventional care was in the child's best interest.[16] A month later, a Massachusetts court considered whether laetrile was an appropriate supplement to chemotherapy for a 3-year-old child with leukemia.[17] Again, both sides presented evidence regarding laetrile's safety and efficacy, but none of the parents' expert witnesses claimed to be experts in blood disease or leukemia.[17] Based on the facts and evidence presented, the Massachusetts court found that using laetrile was not consistent with good medical practice because of the potential adverse interaction with the chemotherapy regimen.[17] The courts in both of these cases were faced with the question of whether a CAM therapy was an appropriate medical treatment under the particular circumstances. Although different types of cancer were at issue, the courts came to two completely different conclusions, based in part on the amount and type of evidence presented at trial about the risks and benefits of the CAM therapy when compared with the conventional treatment options. These decisions highlight the fact-sensitive nature of such inquiries, the importance of expert testimony and medical evidence, and the potential uncertainties of outcome when CAM cases are taken to court. There is, in fact, no case law involving a court's decision regarding the treatment of a psychiatric disorder in a child or adolescent using CAM.

INFORMED CONSENT

To respect an adult patient's personal autonomy and the right to decide what happens to his or her own body, health care professionals are legally and ethically obligated to obtain informed consent from patients before beginning any course of treatment.[9,20] As an example, evidence of informed consent can be shown through chart documentation of verbal consent discussions or through the use of consent forms provided to adult patients. Similar considerations apply to parents of a child with a psychiatric condition. Many clinicians receive verbal rather than written consent from parents for child psychopharmacologic treatments, and place documentation of the consent in the patient's chart; although this is a legally acceptable procedure, it is safer practice from a legal perspective to use an informed consent form signed by the parents, for both routine child psychopharmacologic treatment and CAM treatments.

If consent forms are used they should be tailored to the physician's practice, to the specific therapeutic procedure, and to the particular patient, and should not contain any guarantees. Patient consent forms for CAM treatments should address the following considerations for the patient: any possible benefits and potential complications of the CAM treatment; the availability of any reasonable conventional treatment options; the degree to which the medical literature supports the CAM treatment; the absence of approval by the Food and Drug Administration of the CAM treatment; the patient's express awareness and understanding of known and unknown risks associated with the CAM treatment; and an explanation of why a CAM treatment is being used in lieu of conventional treatment.

Proper documentation of the informed consent process, whether through forms or chart notes, has the added benefit of ensuring that the patient or parent is involved in the decision-making process and has been provided with all the information needed to make an educated decision. Well-documented consent also helps protect the psychiatrist from liability if the patient is injured.[21]

Obtaining informed consent is sometimes more than a discrete event; rather, it may require an ongoing discussion between the psychiatrist, the patient, and the parents.[20] Psychiatrists are required to provide patients/parents with substantive information about the proposed treatment and its risks, benefits, and likely outcomes, as well as alternative courses of action, including nontreatment.[20,22–24] Furthermore, the medical treatment plan should include important medical evidence about the efficacy of each option, whether positive or negative.

In a situation where the psychiatrist recommends a CAM treatment over a viable, established intervention, complete disclosure and proper documentation are paramount. The informed consent disclosures are the same regardless of whether a CAM or conventional therapy is being recommended. The psychiatrist has a legal duty to be forthright about the known risks associated with the CAM therapy and must clearly explain any lack of data or information.[13,24] It is also important for the psychiatrist to make clear that the recommended treatment is outside the norm of conventional medicine. This perspective will require a full discussion of the differences between the alternative and allopathic treatments and why the CAM therapy is being recommended over the conventional treatment, most likely in terms of benefits and risks. As the gatekeeper of information for patients who may be unfamiliar with a CAM treatment, the psychiatrist needs to conduct open and honest dialogue about the treatment, allowing for questions to be asked and concerns to be expressed, before obtaining consent. Because of the heightened liability risks in the event the recommended CAM therapy injures the patient, it is critical for the psychiatrist to document in detail the types of information disclosed as a part of the patient's/parent's consent.

A written consent form is particularly advisable if the parent or child displays any trepidation of the procedure, if they are seemingly resistant to CAM, or if the recommended CAM therapy is risky or lacks published clinical trials supporting its safety and benefits.

Who Can Consent?

Although the law presumes that minors lack the capacity and maturity to make decisions affecting their health, there are certain situations in which minors are legally allowed to make their own treatment decisions, even over parents' preferences. For example, minors who need emergency medical treatment do not need to first obtain parental consent. Similarly, in most states, prior parental consent is not needed for minors who are legally emancipated or are seeking services related to sexual activity, substance abuse, or mental health.[25]

Courts and legislatures have also begun to recognize that some minors possess the competence and maturity to consent to medical treatment, especially as the minor nears adulthood,[26,27] allowing their decisions to supersede their parents' preferences. Studies show that around the age of 14, most adolescents are believed to have developed the cognitive capacity and emotional stability to make their own health care decisions.[28,29] To have the necessary competence to provide informed consent under the law, a person must (1) be able to understand and appreciate the risks and benefits of the proposed treatment and its alternatives, and (2) make the decision voluntarily.[9,24,30] Unless a state's statute or common law provides otherwise, the Mature Minor Doctrine allows unemancipated minors to consent to or refuse general medical treatment if it is clear that they can understand and appreciate the consequences of their action.[30,31] This determination is both legal and factual.

Legally, psychiatrists should be aware of the minor consent laws in their jurisdiction,[30] because these laws differ from state to state. For example, in California there is no provision that allows minors to make health care decisions based on personal maturity,[32] whereas in Alabama, minors aged 14 years and older can consent to any kind of health service, irrespective of whether they have been deemed "mature."[33] The Arkansas legislature has passed a law explicitly incorporating the Mature Minor Doctrine into the consent statute.[34]

In fact, in most jurisdictions the psychiatrist must make the determination of whether the particular child has the maturity necessary to make his or her own treatment decisions. Competence to provide valid consent is situation specific. Psychiatric patients can provide legal consent as long as they possess sufficient decisional capacity for the situation at hand. Factors for the psychiatrist to consider include the minor's age, education, and experience, the risks and benefits of the proposed treatment, and the likely consequences of the decision.[26,30,31,35] The required level of understanding and appreciation will vary with the degree of potential risk involved and the minor's circumstances.[30,31] The psychiatrist should make a more demanding inquiry when the risks associated with the decision are high, such as when a minor is refusing life-preserving treatment. This kind of rigorous evaluation may also be advisable when a minor elects a CAM therapy over a more established, less risky conventional treatment, especially if the patient and parents disagree. However, a mature child or adolescent patient has the right to make an even inadvisable decision regarding a course of treatment as long as (1) the state's statutory or common law recognizes the Mature Minor Doctrine, and (2) the psychiatrist concludes that the patient has the cognitive capacity to make a treatment decision.[30,31] Psychiatrists initially determine whether the patient can consent, but these determinations can be legally challenged, and the court is the final arbiter.[36] Accordingly it is prudent for psychiatrists to create clear treatment and consent notes in the patient's record, especially if the minor is making a risky or controversial decision. It is worth noting that this is rarely an issue in clinical settings. In general, parents make decisions for their child and the youth agrees, even though a mature child or adolescent might legally have the capacity to make the decision.

Even when minors do not have the authority to provide legal consent, it is clinically important to include them in the informed consent discussion by explaining the information to them in a developmentally appropriate way that they can understand and process. The child can then express concerns and beliefs, ask questions, and eventually affirm a desire to accept the treatment plan; this is known as providing "assent."[37] There is no legal duty to obtain minor patients' assent outside of the research context, but from a clinical and ethical point of view the minor's involvement in the decision-making helps move the minor into a treatment alliance with the clinician, increases the patient's understanding and acceptance of the treatment, improves the patient's compliance with treatment, lets patients know that their opinions are valued and valuable, asserts their right to have a say in what happens to them, and ensures that the psychiatrist is responding to the child's thoughts and feelings.[37]

Psychiatrists should seek to obtain assent from minors aged 7 years and older. By age 7, children are generally able to know right from wrong and are able to discuss their motivations and desires. If a CAM treatment is being recommended, the psychiatrist should use clinical judgment to determine whether the youth should be informed about the CAM status of the treatment. For most adolescents, this information may be beneficial to relay, and may prompt the patient to ask important questions or voice concerns. Eliciting a youth's understanding, alliance, and assent may require some clinical approaches not required by the legal requirements of traditional informed consent.

What Satisfies "Informed" Consent?

Two primary standards are used to determine the amount and type of information that must be disclosed before consent is considered valid. The first is the patient-centered standard, which is followed by most US states and requires psychiatrists to disclose all the information a reasonable patient would want to know when deciding whether to consent.[20,23,24] Other states follow the second standard, a profession-centered approach, which only requires disclosing the information a reasonable health care professional would consider appropriate.[23,38] In practice, psychiatrists may have a difficult time determining what treatment alternatives to disclose to satisfy either one of these standards, especially when CAM treatments are taken into consideration. Most courts agree that alternatives that have not been shown to be therapeutically beneficial need to be addressed.[13,39,40] It would be unreasonable to require psychiatrists to be knowledgable about and discuss every possible alternative. Psychiatrists should first make themselves aware of the disclosure standard used in their jurisdictions and then determine whether a reasonable patient would want to know about that treatment alternative, or whether a reasonable health care provider would consider the information appropriate for disclosure. These standards attempt to strike a balance between overloading the patient or parents with too much information, much of which might be unnecessary and confusing, may be overwhelming, and draw out the decision-making process, and, alternatively, divulging too little information, such that the consent is not properly informed. Accordingly the patient-centered standard and profession-centered standard both attempt to arm the patient and parents with sufficient information to make the best decision for the child.

Obligation to Discuss CAM

Over the past few decades, developments in legislative and common law suggest that psychiatrists' disclosure obligations are continuing to evolve.[20,24] At the same time, more and more patients are inquiring about or are already using CAM therapies, either alone or in combination with conventional treatments.[13] This scenario presents both an ethical and legal dilemma: should mental health professionals be required to mention CAM therapies in their discussion of available treatment options during the informed consent process?[41,42]

To date, there have been no recorded legal cases that hold a psychiatrist or other conventional health care provider liable for failing to discuss CAM therapies as an alternative to the proposed treatment plan.[20,40] Accordingly a psychiatrist presumptively has no legal duty to discuss CAM options with patients. Instead, the case law on this subject concerns failure to discuss other conventional alternatives. Thus, when a clinician prescribes a CAM therapy, the clinician should thoroughly advise the patient about established conventional treatments.

Indeed, the general consensus in the legal literature is that there is no obligation to discuss a treatment modality, whether conventional or CAM, that neither has research evidence supporting its efficacy and safety nor has been generally accepted in the medical community.[13,24,40–43] In *Moore v. Baker*, the court considered whether a physician was negligent for failing to mention a particular CAM therapy as an alternative to conventional surgery in treating coronary blockages.[44] The plaintiff presented evidence that some physicians approved its use to treat coronary blockages but, pursuant to Georgia's informed consent statute, the court held that the physician was not liable because chelation therapy was "not generally recognized and accepted in the medical community" as an alternative to coronary surgery.[44] Although some legislatures have articulated standards for disclosing treatment alternatives, it is predominantly up to the courts of each state to determine when a treatment alternative has enough evidence-based research and acceptance to trigger a disclosure obligation. As the body of case law on this matter grows, it will be interesting to look at how willing the courts are to include CAM options in the psychiatrists' disclosure obligations.

In contrast to the *Moore* court's approach, some legal scholars and clinicians argue for a proactive duty to disclose CAM treatments that have shown therapeutic benefits when the information would be material to the patient's decision to consent to or deny conventional treatment; in other words, when a reasonable patient would want to know about the CAM options before making a decision.[20,24,40,45] This scenario requires the psychiatrist to consider the available research data about a particular CAM treatment and make a judgment about whether this information would influence the patient's decision. There is no bright-line test to apply, but disclosure is more likely to affect the patient's decision when there are more data on efficacy and safety.[40,45] When research data are unavailable or inconclusive, the information would likely not be as influential, and there would be no duty to disclose.[20] When there is reliable evidence from research supporting the safety and efficacy of an intervention, even if unconventional, a psychiatrist may have an ethical, and possibly legal, obligation to disclose this option to the patient.[20,24,35] The psychiatrist's disclosure obligation will be expected to expand as the evidence amasses and the medical community starts to embrace the therapy. Until then, however, it is unlikely that a court would hold a psychiatrist liable for not disclosing the CAM therapy as a viable alternative to the recommended treatment.[39,41]

For some CAM treatments, there is strong evidence of safety and efficacy in adults but not in children. As with conventional treatments, it is challenging for clinicians to apply research from adult populations to a child's treatment.[37] From a legal perspective, there is no universally acceptable strategy for dealing with this issue. It is a medical judgment that must be decided on a case-by-case basis.

Even if the psychiatrist does not support the use of CAM, he or she should be aware of relevant research in this area to inform the decision-making process. Regardless of whether the psychiatrist recommends CAM or the patient's parents request CAM, it is good clinical practice for a psychiatrist to be candid about the known risks and benefits.[24,35,40,42] Psychiatrists should inform themselves regarding the evidence base for relevant CAM therapies, using resources such as the articles in this issue. Research suggests that perceived efficacy is the primary reason why most people decide to use CAM.[43] However, it is unlikely a court would find a legal duty for a physician to be knowledgable about a treatment modality that exists primarily outside of mainstream medical practice.

In addition, physicians should know about possible CAM-drug interactions.[44] For example, some studies indicate that certain dietary supplements may diminish or enhance the efficacy of conventional drugs.[45,46] Because most patients do not disclose information about their CAM usage spontaneously, psychiatrists should ask about CAM usage in the history-taking process.[24,47] It is important for the psychiatrist to be aware of all types of treatments being used by the patient so that the psychiatrist is able to structure the treatment plan accordingly and warn the patient of any potential risks.

It has been suggested that the psychiatrist should balance the following 7 factors when deciding whether to support the use of a CAM therapy: (1) severity of the illness; (2) likelihood of response to conventional treatment; (3) adverse effects of conventional treatment; (4) evidence of safety and efficacy of the CAM therapy; (5) degree of understanding of the risks and benefits of the CAM treatment; (6) knowledge and voluntary acceptance of those risks by the patient; and (7) the patient's or parents' commitment to CAM use.[20,24,48] To avoid potential liability, a psychiatrist should not endorse using a CAM therapy that is known to be dangerous or that will interfere with or otherwise divert the child from imminently necessary, conventional care.[13,24,35] The more the evidence base supports the safety and benefits of a particular CAM therapy, the more the psychiatrist should be able to support the parents' decision to use that treatment.[13] Although the decision to use or incorporate a CAM treatment is ultimately up to the patient or patient's parents (provided the decision is not likely, in the view of the prescriber, to result in serious harm to the child),[12] the psychiatrist can have a meaningful role in the decision by educating the family and helping them through the decision-making process, thus ensuring that the parents are making a well-informed decision. In any event, the psychiatrist should continue to monitor the patient on the CAM treatment and, when appropriate, continue conventional treatment.

LIABILITY CONCERNS IN TREATING WITH CAM

Some psychiatrists and other health care professionals have shown trepidation in providing, referring, or recommending CAM out of fear of exposing themselves to liability.[49] By definition, CAM therapies are not the standard of care in conventional medicine, and by departing from the standard of care a psychiatrist may increase the risk of a medical malpractice suit. However, as the evidence base for CAM develops, certain practices gain greater acceptance, and as CAM becomes increasingly integrated into conventional practice, this risk is being minimized. Indeed, CAM is now integrated with conventional care in many medical practices across the country. For example, several University of California (UC) medical campuses have centers for integrative medicine, including UC San Francisco, UC Los Angeles, UC Irvine, and UC San Diego. There is also a growing professional movement for the use of CAM in psychiatry. For instance, there has been a Caucus on Integrative Psychiatry within the American Psychiatric Association since 2004, which has become formalized as the Committee on Alternative and Integrative Medicine. The American Academy of Child and Adolescent Psychiatry also has a Committee on Integrative Medicine.

As one example of how CAM is being integrated with conventional care, a study of older adults with major depression found that the complementary use of Tai Chi augments the use of escitalopram (Lexapro).[50] The study randomized 73 partial responders to escitalopram, who continued to use escitalopram daily, to a 10-week course of either Tai Chi or health education. Subjects in the Tai Chi group were more likely to report greater reduction in depressive symptoms and to achieve a depression remission ($F_{[5, 285]} = 2.26$; $P<.05$). Those subjects also showed greater improvements in health-related quality of life, physical functioning (group $\times$ time interaction: $F_{[1, 66]} = 5.73$; $P = .02$), memory (group $\times$ time interaction: $F_{[1, 65]} = 5.29$; $P<.05$), and a decline in an inflammatory marker, C-reactive protein (time effect: $F_{[2, 78]} = 3.14$, $P<.05$; group $\times$ time trend in posttreatment period: $F_{[1, 39]} = 2.91$;

$P = .10$). Similar findings are emerging in child and adolescent psychiatry, as articles elsewhere in this issue document.

The 2 main types of medical liability are battery and medical malpractice.

Today, battery claims are primarily applicable when a psychiatrist fails to obtain consent before treating a patient[51]; battery claims do not require proof of causation or injury, only that a touching occurred without the patient's consent.[51]

Malpractice claims are more common causes of action. In a medical malpractice claim, liability is imposed when a health care provider's conduct falls below the requisite standard of care and causes harm to the patient. At trial, expert testimony must be presented to establish the standard of care. The standard of care is what an ordinary, prudent professional in the same community would do under similar circumstances.[51,52] Thus, custom plays a central role in determining negligence.[53] However, in rare instances courts will look beyond custom; for example, where a cost-benefit analysis clearly suggests a particular course of action.[54] Such is particularly the case when there is no clear customary standard or when there are multiple schools of thought. Furthermore, for the patient to be successful in a malpractice case, the psychiatrist's negligence must be the cause of the patient's injuries.

Psychiatrists may face liability for practicing integrative medicine (ie, incorporating CAM treatments into their practices), even if the psychiatrist has informed the parents of conventional treatment and has discussed its advantages and disadvantages relative to the CAM treatment, and even if both the parents and physician agreed that the treatment was in the best interest of the child. This situation would require the parents to sue the psychiatrist, alleging that the doctor's negligent action injured their child. For their lawsuit to be successful, a plaintiff's expert witness (generally another child psychiatrist) must state that the treating psychiatrist deviated from the standard of care in providing the CAM treatment, and that providing the CAM treatment was what caused damage to the child. Essentially a physician would then be liable if a judge or jury accepted the testimony of the plaintiff's expert over any potential contradictory defense expert witnesses. A physician has a potential defense in that the parents knowingly and voluntarily assumed the risk of using CAM, but this is not guaranteed to prevent liability.

Disclosure of Risk

Psychiatrists who provide CAM should be aware they may face medical malpractice liability for failure to disclose all of the important known risks involved with a therapy before it is administered, as with conventional care.[13,24,55] Furthermore, a psychiatrist may be held liable for deciding to use CAM when it is contraindicated or when its use is not supported by reliable, scientific evidence, as long as expert testimony given during a trial could establish that an ordinary, prudent professional would not have provided these treatments under similar circumstances.[24,35] Psychiatrists should also be mindful of governing statutes, regulations, and policies that may restrict who can provide certain CAM therapies, because these laws vary depending on the jurisdiction. For example, some states require additional training or an examination for a medical doctor to provide acupuncture.

Referrals to CAM Providers

Another instance whereby psychiatrists may face liability is when making referrals to CAM providers.[56] In general, psychiatrists are not liable for merely referring a patient to another health care provider who then provides substandard care and harms the patient, regardless of whether the referral is to another conventional practitioner or to a CAM specialist.[57,58] Psychiatrists usually are only held liable when they themselves provide the negligent care. However, there are several exceptions.

A psychiatrist may be held directly liable when the referral itself is negligent.[57,58] For example, a referral would be negligent if a psychiatrist failed to treat a patient with suicidal ideation and an active plan, and then referred the patient to a chiropractor. Psychiatrists are freely able to refer patients to other health care providers as long as the referral is reasonable and appropriate under the circumstances.[59,60] Also, a psychiatrist could be subject to liability for referring a patient to a provider whom the psychiatrist knew or should have known was unqualified or provided unsafe care,[57] such as might occur when the psychiatrist knows, or has reason to know, that a specialist may be incompetent.[61] Accordingly, as is the case with a referral to any external provider, it would be prudent for the psychiatrist to perform some due diligence to ascertain whether a CAM provider is properly credentialed, if applicable, and provides proper care. Some CAM providers, such as chiropractors, require state licensure. Others, such as Tai Chi instructors, may not require licensure or even certification. It may be more prudent to recommend an intervention generally rather than a specific provider if no external source of credentialing is available. Alternatively, if a direct referral is made, it should be documented in the patient's record that another physician (especially a CAM-specialized physician) recommended a particular provider.

Direct liability may also be attached if the psychiatrist provides negligent care after the referral is made.[58] For example, referring a patient to a CAM provider should not end the psychiatrist-patient relationship. The psychiatrist should continue to provide appropriate care and monitor the patient to ensure that the alternative therapies are not interfering with the conventional treatment plan or harming the patient. Similarly, if the referral causes a delay in the provision of necessary conventional treatment and the patient is injured as a result, the psychiatrist may face direct medical malpractice liability.[58]

Also, psychiatrists may be held vicariously liable for the negligent acts of others with whom the psychiatrist has a special relationship.[57,62] For example, a setting in which a psychiatrist is likely to be held vicariously liable occurs when the referring psychiatrist supervises or employs the CAM provider, or when the 2 providers engage in a joint undertaking to treat the patient in a collaborative way.[57,58] Although the boundaries of what constitutes a supervisory or collaborative relationship are not always clear, there needs to be some degree of control or intent to integrate treatment efforts on the part of the referring psychiatrist in order for the psychiatrist to be potentially liable for another clinician's actions.[57] For example, a collaborative relationship would likely be identified whereby a psychiatrist's medical practice employed a staff acupuncturist, and a supervisory relationship could be found whereby the psychiatrist dictated the acupuncture points and herbal medicines to be used by the acupuncturist. Simply continuing to treat and monitor patients as they receive CAM therapies from another provider would probably not implicate such a joint relationship. Therefore, vicarious liability is more difficult than direct liability to prove, because the necessary relationship must first be established before the referring psychiatrist can be held liable for the CAM provider's acts.

Disciplinary Action

Psychiatrists should also be aware that they may face professional disciplinary action for providing CAM. For example, the courts upheld a decision in 1985 by the North Carolina Board of Medical Examiners to revoke the license of the only medical doctor openly practicing homeopathy in the state on the sole basis that homeopathy does not conform to the standards of acceptable and prevailing medical practice.[63] This ruling would be less likely today. In fact, after this decision, the North Carolina legislature amended the grounds for discipline to further require that the CAM treatment must have a safety risk greater than the conventional treatment, or that the CAM treatment must be generally ineffective.[64] Texas now has statutory guidelines covering the provision of integrative medicine, which stipulate that physicians shall not be found guilty of unprofessional conduct solely for using CAM, unless it can be demonstrated that such a method has a safety risk for the patient that is unreasonably greater than that of the conventional treatment of the patient's medical condition.[65]

Conventional Medicine Holds the Same Liability as CAM

Having reviewed the principal sources of liability for integrating CAM into a practice, a reader might think that staying as far away from CAM as possible would be prudent. However, conventional medicine raises the same concerns: After reading enough malpractice cases, a physician might decide that it makes no sense for anyone to practice medicine at all. Likewise, patients may think after watching drug advertisements on television, many of which casually mention that death can be a side effect, that no one should ever take medication. Of course, physicians do practice medicine, despite the potential for medical malpractice liability, and patients do take medications, many of which have the potential for serious side effects. The best that can be said of this is that no area of activity is completely free of risk, and that malpractice lawsuits are relatively rare in practice. Liability concerns should not dictate every decision made by a clinician. Ultimately, a physician should practice good medicine and be aware of risks.

SUMMARY

From a legal perspective, any time physicians depart from the customary standard of medical practice they run an increased risk of liability. As CAM by definition refers to practices that have not yet been accepted by the mainstream medical community, it is likely that incorporating CAM practices carries some degree of attendant risk. Despite this, physicians interested in integrating CAM into their practices should be comforted by the lack of malpractice cases regarding the CAM treatment of a psychiatric disorder in a child or adolescent. The reason for the absence of case law is unclear. It may be that CAM treatments are infrequently practiced in child psychiatry and even more rarely in high-risk situations, that this is a practice area with relatively few serious adverse outcomes, that CAM treatments tend to be relatively noninvasive, or that physicians who use CAM generally enjoy less adversarial physician-patient relationships. As long as physicians are knowledgable and mindful of the legal pitfalls relevant to CAM and take appropriate protective action, much as they do when practicing conventional medicine, they should not overestimate the risk of legal liability from judiciously using CAM treatments.

Introducing CAM treatments into a practice is somewhat similar to introducing any new treatment. Most child and adolescent psychiatrists are familiar with these procedures from the use of psychopharmacologic treatments in youth, which were only recently novel treatments, and which still today are often applied clinically before there is a solid database to support their widespread use.

As the delivery of health care continues to evolve into a more integrative approach, psychiatrists may need to make some changes to their daily practice to provide the best possible care to their patients and remain in compliance with the law. The growing popularity of CAM essentially guarantees that all psychiatrists will have to deal with CAM in one way or another. Whether a psychiatrist wants to recommend an alternative therapy or the patient or parents request CAM, the following points will help the psychiatrist provide clinically and legally sound advice.

- CAM can be most safely recommended, from a legal point of view, when there is some published evidence of safety and efficacy. As with conventional treatments, there is no universal standard for when a treatment qualifies as evidence based.
- Any time a CAM treatment is discussed, fully disclose all of the known risks and benefits, so that the patient and the patient's parents can make informed decisions.
- Parents or legal guardians generally have the authority to make health care decisions on their children's behalf, although there are situations whereby the youth's decision may have precedence. All treatment decisions should be made in the child's best interest. If the parents' decision to use a CAM treatment is likely to subject the child to serious harm, the psychiatrist is legally obligated to notify welfare authorities.
- Only refer patients to CAM providers who are properly trained, and credentialed if applicable, and continue to monitor and treat the patient with conventional care as needed.
- Document any discussion of CAM in the medical record. If the parent insists on a therapy against medical advice, make clear documentation in the medical record of the parent's voluntary and knowing assumption of the risk.
- As evidence emerges that a CAM therapy may be safe and effective, or as a therapy gains widespread acceptance, there may be an obligation to disclose it as a viable treatment alternative to conventional treatment.

REFERENCES

1. Abbott RB. Treating the health care crisis: complementary and alternative medicine for PPACA. DePaul J Health Care Law 2012;14:35.
2. Abbott RB, Hui KK, Hays RD, et al. Medical student attitudes toward complementary, alternative, and integrative medicine. Evid Based Complement Alternat Med 2011;2011:985243.
3. Cohen M. Complementary & alternative medicine legal boundaries and regulatory perspectives. Baltimore (MD): Johns Hopkins University Press; 1998. p. 4–8, xii.
4. Davis M, Darden P. Use of complementary and alternative medicine by children in the United States. Arch Pediatr Adolesc Med 2003;157:393–6.
5. Parham v J.R., 442 U.S. 584, 602–06 (1979).
6. Boozang K. CAM for kids. Houst J Health Law Policy 2001;1:109–32.
7. Rosato JL. Using bioethics discourse to determine when parents should make health care decisions for their children. Temple Law Rev 2000;73:1–68.
8. Gilmour J, Harrison C, Cohen M, et al. Considering complementary and alternative medicine alternatives in cases of life-threatening illness: applying the best-interests test. Pediatrics 2011;128:S175–80.
9. Redding R. Children's competence to provide informed consent for mental health treatment. Wash Lee Law Rev 1993;50:695–751.
10. American Medical Association. Pediatric Decision-Making: Report of the Council on Ethical and Judicial Affairs. CEJA Report 8–1–07. Available at: http://www.ama-assn.org/doc/code-medical-ethics/10016a.pdf.

11. Eve v Mrs E, 31 DLR (4th) 1 (SCC 1986).
12. Black L. Limiting parents' rights in medical decision-making. Virtual Mentor 2006;8:676–80.
13. Cohen M, Kemper K. Complementary therapies in pediatrics: a legal perspective. Pediatrics 2005;115:774–80.
14. Prince v Massachusetts, 321 U.S. 158, 170 (1944).
15. Renfro v Fehrmann, 817 S.W.2d 592 (Mo. Ct. App. 1991).
16. In the Matter of Joseph Hofbauer, 393 N.E.2d 1009 (N.Y. 1979).
17. Custody of a Minor, 393 N.E.2d 836 (Mass. 1979).
18. Richards EP, Rathbun KC. Medical care law. Gaithersburg, VA: Aspen Publishing Company; 1999.
19. Cohen M. A fixed star in health care reform: the emerging paradigm of holistic healing. Ariz State Law J 1995;27:79–172.
20. Gilmour J, Harrison C, Cohen M, et al. Informed consent: advising patients and parents about complementary and alternative medicine therapies. Pediatrics 2011;128:S187–92.
21. Vincler L, Nicol M. When ignorance isn't bliss: what healthcare practitioners and facilities should know about complementary and alternative medicine. J Health Law 1997;30:160.
22. Truman v Thomas, 27 Cal.3d 285 (Cal. 1980).
23. Canterbury v Spence, 464 F.2d 772 (D.C. Cir. 1972).
24. Verhoef M, Boon H, Page S. Talking to cancer patients about complementary therapies: is it the physician's responsibility? Curr Oncol 2008;15: s88–93.
25. Boonstra H, Nash E. Minors and the right to consent to health care. Issues Brief (Alan Guttmacher Inst) 2000;2:1–6.
26. Belcher v Charleston Area Medical Ctr., 188 W.Va. 105 (W.Va. 1992).
27. Miss. Code Ann.§ 41-41-3(h).
28. Alderson P. Competent children? minor's consent to health care treatment and research. Soc Sci Med 2007;65:2272–83.
29. Weithorn L, Campbell S. The competency of children and adolescents to make informed decisions. Child Dev 1982;53:1589–98.
30. Gilmour J, Harrison C, Cohen M, et al. Treating teens: considerations when adolescents want to use complementary and alternative medicine. Pediatrics 2011;128:S161–6.
31. Derish M, Heuvel K. Mature minors should have the right to refuse life-sustaining medical treatment. J Law Med Ethics 2000;28:109–24.
32. English A, Kenney K. State minor consent laws: a summary. 2nd edition. Chappel Hill, NC: Center for Adolescent Health and the Law; 2003.
33. Ala. Code § 22-8-4.
34. Ark. Code § 20-9-602.
35. In re E.G., 549 N.E.2d 322 (Ill. 1989).
36. Gilmour J, Harrison C, Asadi L, et al. Childhood immunization: when physicians and parents disagree. Pediatrics 2011;128(Suppl 4):S167–74.
37. Popper CW. Medical unknowns and ethical consent: prescribing psychotropic medication for children in the face of uncertainty. In: Popper CW, editor. Psychiatric pharmacosciences of children and adolescents. Washington, DC: American Psychiatric Press; 1987. p. 127–61.
38. Robinson v Bleicher, 559 N.W.2d 473 (Neb. 1997) (disapproved of on other grounds in Hamilton v. Bares, 678 N.W.2d 74 (Neb. 2004)).
39. Morris v. Ferriss, 669 So.2d 1316 (La. App. 1996).

40. Weir M. Obligation to advise of options for treatment—medical doctors and complementary and alternative medicine practitioners. J Law Med 2003;10:296–307.
41. Vohra S, Cohen MH. Ethics of complementary and alternative medicine use in children. Pediatr Clin North Am 2007;54(6):875–84.
42. Cohen MH, Kemper KJ, Stevens L, et al. Pediatric use of complementary therapies: ethical and policy choices. Pediatrics 2005;116(4):e568–75.
43. Knoll A. The reawakening of complementary and alternative medicine at the turn of the twenty-first century: filling the void in conventional biomedicine. J Contemp Health Law Policy 2004;20:329–66.
44. Moore v Baker, US Dist LEXIS 14712 (S.D.Ga. 1991) (aff'd, 989 F.2d 1129, 1132 (11th Cir. 1993)).
45. Ernst E, Cohen M. Informed consent in complementary and alternative medicine. Arch Intern Med 2001;161:2288–92.
46. Plumber v State, 634 So.2d 1347 (La. Ct. App. 1994).
47. Caulfield T. Physicians, alternative medicine and the duty of informed consent. Health Ethics Today 2000;11:3.
48. Astin J. Why patients use alternative medicine. JAMA 1998;279:1548–53.
49. Gilmour J, Harrison C, Asadi L, et al. Natural health product-drug interactions: evolving responsibilities to take complementary and alternative medicine into account. Pediatrics 2011;128(Suppl 4):S155–60.
50. Goldman R, Rogovik A, Lai D, et al. Potential interactions of drug-natural health products and natural health products-natural health products among children. J Pediatr 2008;152:521–6.
51. Cvijovic K, Boon H, Barnes J, et al. A tool for rapid identification of potential herbal medicine drug interactions. Can Pharm J 2009;142:224–7.
52. Eisenberg D. Advising patients who seek alternative medical therapies. Ann Intern Med 1997;127:61–9.
53. Cramm T, Hartz A, Green M. Ascertaining customary care in malpractice cases: asking those who know. Wake Forest Law Rev 2002;37:699–700.
54. Helling v. Carey, 519 P.2d 981 (Wash. 1974).
55. Adams K, Cohen M, Eisenberg D, et al. Ethical considerations of complementary and alternative medical therapies in conventional medical settings. Ann Intern Med 2002;137:660–4.
56. Gilmour J, Harrison C, Cohen MH, et al. Pediatric use of complementary and alternative medicine: legal, ethical, and clinical issues in decision-making. Pediatrics 2011;128(Suppl 4):S149–54.
57. Lavretsky H, Alstein LL, Olmstead RE, et al. Complementary use of tai chi chih augments escitalopram treatment of geriatric depression: a randomized controlled trial. Am J Geriatr Psychiatry 2011;19:839–50.
58. Blanchard v Kellum, 975 S.W.2d 522 (Tenn. 1998).
59. Peters P. The quiet demise of deference to custom: malpractice law at the millennium. Wash Lee Law Rev 2000;57:163–205.
60. Clark v Dept. of Professional Regulation, 463 So.2d 328 (Fla. Dist. Ct. App. 1985).
61. Estate of Tranor v. Bloomsburg Hospital, 60 F.Supp.2d 412 (M.D. Penn. 1999).
62. Gilmour J, Harrison C, Asadi L, et al. Referrals and shared or collaborative care: managing relationships with complementary and alternative medicine practitioners. Pediatrics 2011;128(Suppl 4):S181–6.
63. In re Guess, 327 N.C. 46 (N.C. 1990).
64. N.C. Gen. Stat. § 90–14(a)(6).
65. 22 Tex. Admin. Code § 200.3 (2013).

Building an Evidence Base in Complementary and Integrative Healthcare for Child and Adolescent Psychiatry

Emmeline Edwards, PhD[a],*, David Mischoulon, MD, PhD[b],
Mark Rapaport, MD[c], Barbara Stussman, BA[d],
Wendy Weber, ND, PhD, MPH[a]

KEYWORDS

- Complementary medicine • Integrative medicine • Mind and body
- Natural products • Child and adolescent psychiatry • Manipulative therapies
- CAM research • Epidemiology

KEY POINTS

- The integration of safe and efficacious complementary therapies with proven conventional medicine may result in better patient outcomes as assessed by symptom relief, school performance, social functioning, and family/peer relations.
- The evidence for complementary therapies in child and adolescent psychiatry is fragmentary, with a paucity of well-designed, adequately powered clinical trials incorporating suitable controls on promising modalities (mind and body, manipulative, natural products).
- The National Center for Complementary and Alternative Medicine third strategic plan, *Exploring the Science of Complementary and Alternative Medicine* (http://nccam.nih. gov/about/plans/2011), strongly emphasizes building the evidence base for complementary and integrative approaches, using a personalized, individualized decision-making process about the use of complementary therapies.

Disclaimer/Conflict of Interest: The views expressed in this article are those of the authors and are not necessarily those of the National Center for Complementary and Alternative Medicine at the National Institutes of Health, US Department of Health and Human Services. The authors have no known conflicts of interest.
[a] Division of Extramural Research, National Center for Complementary and Alternative Medicine (NCCAM), National Institutes of Health, 6707 Democracy Boulevard, Suite 401, Bethesda, MD 20892, USA; [b] Depression Clinical and Research Program, Massachusetts General Hospital, Harvard Medical School, 1 Bowdoin Square, 6th Floor, Boston, MA 02114, USA; [c] Department of Psychiatry and Behavioral Sciences, Emory University School of Medicine, 201 Dowman Drive, Atlanta, GA 30322, USA; [d] National Center for Complementary and Alternative Medicine (NCCAM), National Institutes of Health, 6707 Democracy Boulevard, Suite 401, Bethesda, MD 20892, USA
* Corresponding author.
E-mail address: edwardse@mail.nih.gov

Child Adolesc Psychiatric Clin N Am 22 (2013) 509–529
http://dx.doi.org/10.1016/j.chc.2013.03.007
1056-4993/13/$ – see front matter Published by Elsevier Inc.
childpsych.theclinics.com

INTRODUCTION/BACKGROUND
Definition of Complementary and Integrative Health Care

Complementary and integrative health care includes a range of therapeutic approaches.[1] The National Center for Complementary and Alternative Medicine (NCCAM), within the National Institutes of Health (NIH), defines these health care strategies as "a group of diverse medical and health care systems, practices, and products that are not generally considered part of conventional medicine" (http://nccam.nih. gov/health/whatiscam/).[2] Many of these treatments are aimed at promoting health by promoting overall well-being, but some interventions have been examined for their value in treating certain disorders or targeting specific symptoms.

Based on the research methodological approaches needed to best study the effects, complementary medicine research falls into 2 basic categories: natural products and mind and body intervention research. Natural product therapies encompass a variety of herbal medicines (botanicals), probiotics, vitamins, minerals, other natural products, as well as diet-based therapies. Mind and body therapies include practices that focus on interactions among the mind/brain, body, and behavior (eg, meditation, biofeedback, deep breathing exercises, guided imagery, progressive relaxation, hypnotherapy, yoga, qi gong, tai chi), as well as approaches that entail procedures on bodily structures or systems performed by a therapist (eg, chiropractic or osteopathic spinal manipulation, massage therapy, acupuncture).

Complementary and Integrative Health Care Modalities in Child and Adolescent Psychiatry

Space constraints preclude an exhaustive review of the literature. This article provides an overview of complementary and integrative modalities that, based on data from the 2007 National Health Interview Survey (NHIS), are widely used in the United States by families in which children have mental health diagnoses. The most commonly used complementary and integrative strategies for child and adolescent psychiatry fall into the categories of natural products, mind and body approaches, and manipulative and body-based practices. For example, half of families of children with autism spectrum disorder reported use by the child of 1 or more natural products; 30%, a mind-body therapy; and 25%, a manipulation or body-based method.[3]

This article focuses on clinical conditions that are difficult to manage solely with conventional medicine, citing review articles and meta-analyses for a more in-depth review of specific areas of interest. Where the research evidence supports use of complementary approaches, where the research is weak, and where further research is needed to test safety and efficacy are described.

Historical Evolution

Over the past 20 years, there has been a dramatic increase in the prevalence and severity of psychiatric disorders in childhood and adolescence, with significant impairment in functioning and disruption of psychosocial development. This situation has led, with the goal of intervening early, to the increased use of psychotropic medication treatments in the pediatric population.[3,4] For some stakeholders, the increased use of medication of children seems justified, given how rapidly change occurs during childhood and the long-term impact on development if the youth's psychiatric symptoms remain unabated. However, there have been increasing concerns about potentially severe adverse effects of mental health drugs, such as possible suicidality with antidepressants and anticonvulsants,[5] addiction potential of stimulants, as well as commonly used antidepressants and antianxiety agents[6]; metabolic syndrome, weight gain, and gynecomastia[7] with antipsychotics, and sudden death in pediatric as well as adult patients on antidepressants and stimulants.[8]

Consequently, the psychiatric community has increased its interest in understanding the efficacy, safety, and patterns of use of complementary and integrative strategies. Parents of children with mental health conditions have also shown increasing interest in these treatments, as the caregivers' role in treatment-related planning and decision making has evolved from ally to full partner to driver[9]: for example, 15% of children being treated for a psychiatric disorder in community mental health centers had been administered herbal products by their primary caregivers within the previous year.

Similarly, various evidence-based mind-body approaches are being incorporated in the care of children with mental health disorders. Meditation practice, particularly mindfulness meditation (moment-to-moment nonjudgmental awareness of breathing, physical sensations, emotions, and thoughts), can change brain activation patterns and contribute to enhanced mood, reduced anxiety, improved stress management, reduced pain, and enhanced immune function.[10] Mindfulness techniques applied in a Boston public middle school resulted in improvement of various measures, including general well-being.[11] Movement-based meditation, including yoga, tai chi, and qi gong, has also been assessed as potential strategies for treating anxiety and depression.[12,13] In addition, several small studies have suggested that relaxation may assist in treating phobias or panic disorder. Relaxation therapy was found, in a small randomized controlled trial (RCT), to be as effective as cognitive behavioral therapy (a well-researched, evidence-based treatment) for a group of 30 depressed adolescents.[14] Although this is an area of active investigation, there are no data from large-scale, high-quality RCTs. Similarly, there are no conclusive studies on the effect of acupuncture in the treatment of mental disorders.[15]

Historically, there has been expanding research on and clinical use of a variety of complementary and integrative modalities for treating psychiatric disorders in youth, but the research database remains sparse compared with the widespread use by consumers.

COMPLEMENTARY AND INTEGRATIVE MODALITIES IN CHILD AND ADOLESCENT PSYCHIATRY
Demographics of Complementary Therapy Use

The statistics shown in **Tables 1–3** are based on data from the 2007 NHIS; specifically, the components of the Adult and Child Complementary and Alternative Medicine supplements, the Sample Adult core, the Sample Child core, and the Family core.[16] These analyses were performed separately for children ages 0 to 17 years and 18 to 21 years, and direct comparisons between these 2 age groups are not possible for 2 reasons. First, separate questionnaires were used for each, and the specific items were worded differently. Second, information for children aged 0 to 17 years is reported by the child's parent or guardian, whereas information for youth aged 18 to 21 years is self-reported; research has shown that information provided by proxy respondents is not equivalent to that reported by children and adolescents with behavioral and emotional problems.[16] Consistent with other studies,[17] use of vitamin and mineral supplements was not included in total complementary medicine use, but is shown separately in the Tables.

Tables 1 and **2** show sociodemographic factors for children who used complementary therapies within the previous 12 months. Consistent with previous research,[17,18] factors associated with use of complementary therapies in children include being

Table 1
Complementary therapy use among US children aged 0 to 17 years in the past 12 months, 2007 NHIS

	All Complementary Therapies[a]		Biologically Based Therapies[b]		Mind-Body Therapies[c]		Manipulative and Body-Based Therapies[d]		Vitamin and Mineral Supplements[e]	
	Number (in Thousands)	Percent (Standard Error)	Number (in Thousands)	Percent (Standard Error)	Number (in Thousands)	Percent (Standard Error)	Number (in Thousands)	Percent (Standard Error)	Number (in Thousands)	Percent (Standard Error)
Total[f]	7760	10.5 (0.44)	3790	5.1 (0.34)	3121	4.2 (0.29)	2678	3.6 (0.27)	31,377	42.6 (0.72)
Therapy Used to Treat Health Problem[g]										
Used to treat a specific health problem	3152	4.3 (0.29)	1420	1.9 (0.24)	828	1.1 (0.15)	1341	1.8 (0.17)	1102	1.5 (0.16)
Not used to treat a specific health problem	3721	5.0 (0.3)	1235	1.7 (0.17)	2293	3.1 (0.24)	1337	1.8 (0.19)	25,173	34.1 (0.7)
Sex										
Male	3735	9.9 (0.62)	1957	5.2 (0.52)	1393	3.7 (0.43)	1189	3.2 (0.33)	15,852	42.1 (0.96)
Female	4025	11.2 (0.56)	1833	5.1 (0.43)	1728	4.8 (0.35)	1489	4.1 (0.39)	15,525	43.1 (1.01)
Age										
0–4 y	1268	6.2 (0.59)	762	3.7 (0.47)	383	1.9 (0.33)	436	2.1 (0.39)	7766	37.7 (1.19)
5–11 y	2691	9.6 (0.66)	1370	4.9 (0.52)	1062	3.8 (0.40)	781	2.8 (0.38)	14,133	50.6 (1.12)
12–17 y	3801	15.1 (0.79)	1658	6.6 (0.61)	1677	6.6 (0.61)	1461	5.8 (0.5)	9478	37.6 (1.11)
Race										
White, single race	6482	11.6 (0.52)	3184	5.7 (0.41)	2440	4.4 (0.35)	2431	4.4 (0.33)	24,997	44.9 (0.82)
Black or African American, single race	501	4.4 (0.62)	183	1.6 (0.35)	322	2.8 (0.54)	83	0.7 (0.25)[i]	3760	32.9 (1.4)
Ethnicity										
Hispanic	928	6.0 (0.58)	465	3.0 (0.44)	403	2.6 (0.38)	276	1.8 (0.34)	4859	31.7 (1.06)
Non-Hispanic	6832	11.7 (0.54)	3325	5.7 (0.42)	2718	4.7 (0.35)	2402	4.1 (0.33)	26,518	45.4 (0.86)

Family Structure										
Mother and father	5995	11.5 (0.55)	3025	5.8 (0.45)	2166	4.1 (0.34)	2153	4.1 (0.34)	23,728	45.4 (0.83)
Mother, no father	1395	8.2 (0.75)	573	3.4 (0.48)	800	4.7 (0.6)	423	2.5 (0.37)	6226	36.8 (1.38)
Parent's Education										
Less than high school diploma	340	3.8 (0.66)	124	1.4 (0.41)	163	1.8 (0.45)	128	1.4 (0.48)[i]	1920	21.2 (1.35)
High school diploma or General Educational Development	1060	6.6 (0.68)	470	2.9 (0.49)	365	2.3 (0.39)	405	2.5 (0.43)	5264	32.9 (1.26)
More than high school	6207	13.5 (0.61)	3127	6.8 (0.5)	2532	5.5 (0.42)	2108	4.6 (0.37)	23,475	51.2 (0.88)
Poverty Status[h]										
Poor	622	5.3 (0.7)	267	2.3 (0.46)	343	2.9 (0.46)	160	1.4 (0.35)	3177	26.9 (1.36)
Near poor	1201	7.8 (0.86)	678	4.4 (0.69)	343	2.2 (0.5)	402	2.6 (0.48)	5810	38.0 (1.57)
Not poor	5444	13.9 (0.68)	2645	6.8 (0.54)	2245	5.7 (0.45)	1944	5.0 (0.41)	19,932	51.0 (0.94)
Health Insurance										
Private	5561	12.8 (0.6)	2603	6.0 (0.47)	2221	5.1 (0.41)	2078	4.8 (0.4)	21,653	49.7 (0.92)
Public	1583	6.7 (0.6)	804	3.4 (0.42)	704	3.0 (0.42)	435	1.9 (0.3)	7617	32.4 (1.16)
Uninsured	594	9.3 (1.22)	372	5.8 (1.13)	191	3.0 (0.55)	160	2.5 (0.65)	2052	32.0 (1.89)
Region										
Northeast	1469	11.9 (1.19)	614	5.0 (0.83)	669	5.4 (0.75)	492	4.0 (0.82)	5558	45.0 (2.1)
Midwest	2098	12.0 (0.97)	887	5.1 (0.61)	778	4.5 (0.66)	781	4.5 (0.57)	8158	46.8 (1.44)
South	2029	7.5 (0.59)	1051	3.9 (0.46)	759	2.8 (0.35)	646	2.4 (0.32)	10,885	40.0 (1.12)
West	2164	12.9 (0.94)	1237	7.4 (0.92)	915	5.5 (0.68)	759	4.5 (0.6)	6777	40.5 (1.49)
Family Member Reporting										
Parent uses complementary therapies	3003	23.4 (1.37)	1485	11.6 (1.12)	1267	9.9 (0.41)	984	7.7 (0.83)	7471	58.1 (1.66)

(continued on next page)

Table 1
(continued)

	All Complementary Therapies[a]		Biologically Based Therapies[b]		Mind-Body Therapies[c]		Manipulative and Body-Based Therapies[d]		Vitamin and Mineral Supplements[e]	
	Number (in Thousands)	Percent (Standard Error)	Number (in Thousands)	Percent (Standard Error)	Number (in Thousands)	Percent (Standard Error)	Number (in Thousands)	Percent (Standard Error)	Number (in Thousands)	Percent (Standard Error)
Parent does not use complementary therapies	897	3.8 (0.47)	306	1.3 (0.19)	386	1.6 (0.38)	270	1.1 (0.23)	8421	35.2 (1.04)
Other relative or nonrelative uses complementary therapies	90	17.7 (4.29)	44	8.7 (3.46)	59	11.7 (3.38)	31	6.1 (2.63)[i]	217	42.6 (6.68)
Other relative or nonrelative does not use complementary therapies	54	3.2 (1.15)	j	j	j	j	j	j	353	21.3 (2.77)

[a] Includes NVNMDS (nonvitamin, nonmineral, dietary supplements), special diets, homeopathy, biofeedback, relaxation techniques (meditation, guided imagery, progressive relaxation, and deep breathing), yoga, tai chi, qi gong, chiropractic and osteopathic manipulation, massage, movement therapies (Feldenkrais, Alexander technique, Pilates, and Trager).

[b] Includes NVNMDS, special diets, and homeopathy.

[c] Includes biofeedback, relaxation techniques, hypnosis, and yoga, tai chi, and qi gong.

[d] Includes chiropractic or osteopathic manipulation, massage, and movement therapies.

[e] Includes multivitamin or mineral combination, calcium, chromium, coral calcium, folic acid/folate, iron, magnesium, niacin, potassium, selenium, vitamin A, vitamin B complex, vitamin B_6, vitamin B_{12}, vitamin C, vitamin D, vitamin E, vitamin K, zinc, and vitamin packets.

[f] Total complementary therapy use is less than total of individual categories because some respondents used multiple therapies.

[g] Treat variable totals do not equal totals for other variables because reference period for this item for NVNMDS and vitamins was past 30 days rather than past 12 months as for all other therapies.

[h] Poverty status is based on family income and family size using the Census Bureau's poverty thresholds for 2006. Poor is defined as below the poverty threshold. Near poor persons have incomes of 100% to less than 200% of the poverty threshold. Not poor persons have incomes 200% or greater than the poverty threshold.

[i] Estimate has a relative standard error of greater than 30% and less than or equal to 50% and does not meet the standard of reliability or precision.

[j] Estimate has a relative standard error greater than 50% and is not shown.

older, white, of non-Hispanic origin, having a parent with higher education, of higher income (poverty status), not living in the south, and having a parent who used complementary therapies. In addition, for children 18 to 21 years old, being female was associated with greater use of complementary therapies, whereas having public health insurance was associated with less use of these therapies. These trends held across the major categories of complementary medicine: biologically based, mind and body, manipulative and body-based, and vitamin and mineral supplements, except that 5-year-old to 11-year-old children are more likely to take vitamins than children in the other age groups, consistent with previous research.[19]

Intended Use of Complementary Therapy

The 2007 NHIS included a question to assess whether children who used complementary therapies did so to treat a specific health problem or condition ("Yes" or "No"), rather than for other reasons, such as to promote general health. Overall, in both age groups (0–17 years and 18–21 years), most youths used complementary therapies for reasons other than to treat a specific health problem, especially with the mind and body therapies (see **Tables 1** and **2**). Although we were unable to find similar studies in children, our findings are consistent with Davis and colleagues,[20] who found that adults use mind and body therapies more than any other category of complementary medicine for reasons other than specific medical treatment. Vitamin and mineral supplements, not included in the total complementary medicine category, are rarely used to treat specific disorders in youngsters of both age groups (see **Tables 1** and **2**).

We also examined use of complementary therapies in 0-year-old to 21-year-old children for 5 mental health conditions: anxiety/phobia or fears, insomnia or trouble sleeping, attention-deficit/hyperactivity disorder (ADHD), depression, and autism. Use rates for these conditions are similar to those found in other publications.[21–26] For both age groups, children with these 5 psychiatric conditions are more likely to use complementary therapies than all children their age (ie, children with and without these mental health conditions). This finding is consistent with previous studies reporting higher use of complementary medicine among children with medical conditions.[17,27–29] Likewise, children with mental health conditions were more likely to take vitamin supplements than all children. In both age groups, children who had anxiety, phobia, or fears were twice as likely to use complementary therapies compared with all children their age. For children with insomnia or trouble sleeping, and for children with autism, similarly high rates of complementary medicine use were found. Children with ADHD and depression were also considerably more likely to use complementary therapies than all children, but at lower rates than found for anxiety/phobia/fears, insomnia/trouble sleeping, and autism. Thus, although youths generally used complementary interventions for reasons other than treating specific conditions, youths with psychiatric and other medical conditions tended to use more complementary interventions than other youths.

NCCAM Research Priorities for Natural Products

The NCCAM third strategic plan, *Exploring the Science of Complementary and Alternative Medicine* (http://nccam.nih.gov/about/plans/2011),[1] emphasizes the importance of building the evidence base for complementary and integrative approaches, especially for personalized, individualized decision making. As part of this strategy, NCCAM places a strong emphasis on basic mechanism-oriented research, especially exploratory studies that have the potential to yield mechanistic insights, and to identify biological signals of physiologic effects. The goal is a sufficient level of mechanistic insight to allow measurement of signatures of biological effects relevant to coherent

Table 2
Complementary therapy use among US children aged 18 to 21 years in the past 12 months, 2007 NHIS

	All Complementary Therapies[a]		Biologically Based Therapies[b]		Mind-Body Therapies[c]		Manipulative and Body-Based Therapies[d]		Vitamin and Mineral Supplements[e]	
	Number (in Thousands)	Percent (Standard Error)	Number (in Thousands)	Percent (Standard Error)	Number (in Thousands)	Percent (Standard Error)	Number (in Thousands)	Percent (Standard Error)	Number (in Thousands)	Percent (Standard Error)
Total[f]	4495	27.5 (1.72)	1829	11.2 (1.13)	2849	17.4 (1.4)	1679	10.3 (1.12)	6654	40.7 (2.06)
Therapy Used to Treat Health Problem[g]										
Used to treat a specific health problem	1197	7.3 (0.87)	304	1.9 (0.45)	368	2.2 (0.51)	698	4.3 (0.73)	392	2.4 (0.53)
Not used to treat a specific health problem	3003	18.4 (1.48)	799	4.9 (0.66)	2482	15.2 (1.29)	982	6.0 (0.93)	4169	25.5 (1.66)
Sex										
Male	1789	21.9 (2.1)	737	9.0 (1.5)	1127	13.8 (1.88)	613	7.5 (1.23)	2826	34.6 (2.94)
Female	2707	33.0 (2.45)	1092	13.3 (1.67)	1722	21.0 (2.09)	1067	13.0 (1.79)	3827	46.7 (2.65)
Race										
White, single race	3480	30.0 (2.1)	1453	12.5 (1.46)	2128	18.3 (1.78)	1395	12.0 (1.45)	4922	42.4 (2.49)
Black or African American, single race	514	20.1 (3.27)	164	6.4 (1.95)	366	14.3 (2.77)	188	7.3 (2.32)	935	36.6 (4.12)
Ethnicity										

Hispanic	402	14.2 (2.37)	118	4.2 (1.32)	293	10.4 (1.88)	100	3.5 (1.16)	748	26.5 (3.08)
Non-Hispanic	4094	30.2 (1.91)	1711	12.6 (1.32)	2556	18.9 (1.62)	1579	11.7 (1.33)	5905	43.6 (2.37)
Poverty Status[h]										
Poor	1417	32.2 (2.64)	586	13.3 (1.71)	899	20.4 (2.19)	459	10.4 (1.89)	1910	43.4 (3.93)
Near poor	535	20.8 (3.49)	197	7.7 (1.9)	358	13.9 (3.15)	184	7.1 (2.11)	944	36.7 (4.63)
Not poor	2085	28.3 (2.87)	859	11.7 (1.96)	1390	18.9 (2.37)	827	11.2 (1.95)	3015	41.0 (3.01)
Health Insurance										
Private	2999	31.0 (2.34)	1199	12.4 (1.58)	1889	19.5 (1.97)	1280	13.2 (1.72)	4550	47.1 (2.88)
Public	454	19.8 (3.27)	194	8.5 (2.12)	270	11.8 (2.53)	151	6.6 (2.03)	708	30.9 (3.63)
Uninsured	983	23.2 (2.8)	418	9.8 (2.02)	649	15.3 (2.42)	235	5.5 (1.54)	1334	31.4 (3.24)
Region										
Northeast	835	31.4 (4.73)	350	13.2 (3.39)	563	21.2 (3.8)	238	8.9 (2.5)	1021	38.4 (7.57)
Midwest	1251	34.6 (3.51)	418	11.6 (2.52)	712	19.7 (2.36)	543	15.0 (2.75)	1589	44.0 (3.07)
South	1252	21.0 (2.62)	563	9.5 (1.62)	752	12.6 (2.26)	338	5.7 (1.11)	2405	40.4 (3.51)
West	1157	28.0 (3.44)	497	12.0 (2.21)	823	19.9 (3.03)	561	13.6 (2.76)	1638	39.6 (3.34)

a Includes NVNMDS (nonvitamin, no-mineral, dietary supplements), special diets, homeopathy, biofeedback, relaxation techniques (meditation, guided imagery, progressive relaxation, and deep breathing), yoga, tai chi, qi gong, chiropractic and osteopathic manipulation, massage, movement therapies (Feldenkrais, Alexander technique, Pilates, and Trager).

b Includes NVNMDS, special diets, and homeopathy.

c Includes biofeedback, relaxation techniques, hypnosis, and yoga, tai chi, and qi gong.

d Includes chiropractic or osteopathic manipulation, massage, and movement therapies.

e Includes multivitamin or mineral combination, calcium, chromium, coral calcium, folic acid/folate, iron, magnesium, niacin, potassium, selenium, vitamin A, vitamin B complex, vitamin B_6, vitamin B_{12}, vitamin C, vitamin D, vitamin E, vitamin K, zinc, and vitamin packets.

f Total complementary therapy use is less than total of individual categories because some respondents used multiple therapies.

g Treat variable totals do not equal totals for other variables because reference period for this item for NVNMDS and vitamins was past 30 days rather than past 12 months as for all other therapies.

h Poverty status is based on family income and family size using the Census Bureau's poverty thresholds for 2006. Poor is defined as below the poverty threshold. Near poor persons have incomes of 100% to less than 200% of the poverty threshold. Not poor persons have incomes 200% or greater than the poverty threshold.

Table 3
Children aged 0 to 21 years with selected health conditions who used complementary therapies in the past 12 months, 2007 NHIS

	Children with Selected Conditions[a]		Children with Selected Conditions Who Used Complementary Therapies[b,c]		Children Who Used Complementary Therapies for Selected Conditions[d]		Children with Selected Conditions Who Used Vitamin and Mineral Supplements[e,f]	
	Number (in Thousands)	Percent (Standard Error)	Number (in Thousands)	Percent (Standard Error)	Number (in Thousands)	Percent (Standard Error)	Number (in Thousands)	Percent (Standard Error)
Anxiety/Phobia or Fears								
0–4 y[g]	106	2.5 (0.76)[j]	33	31.0 (13.77)[j]	k	k	76	71.9 (14.44)
5–11 y[g]	2184	7.8 (0.59)	584	26.8 (3.86)	197	33.7 (7.77)	1291	59.1 (3.81)
12–17 y[g]	2814	11.2 (0.66)	922	32.8 (3.19)	144	15.6 (3.78)	1318	46.8 (3.51)
18–21 y[h]	1591	9.7 (0.99)	1591	49.3 (5.32)	118	15.0 (5.55)[j]	862	54.2 (5.4)
Insomnia or Trouble Sleeping								
0–4 y[g]	192	2.3 (0.54)	70	36.5 (12.49)[j]	k	k	88	45.7 (11.77)
5–11 y[g]	1070	3.8 (0.41)	214	20.0 (4.07)	53	24.9 (9.83)[j]	596	55.7 (5.34)
12–17 y[g]	1912	7.6 (0.57)	575	30.1 (3.41)	64	11.1 (3.52)[j]	838	43.8 (4.19)
18–21 y[g]	1761	10.8 (1.0)	793	45.0 (5.36)	k	k	890	50.5 (5.47)
Attention-Deficit/Hyperactivity Disorder–Attention-Deficit Disorder								
0–4 y[i]	179	1.4 (0.41)		k	k	k	119	66.2 (15.2)
5–11 y[i]	1644	5.9 (0.44)	238	14.5 (2.54)	76	31.9 (8.94)	788	47.9 (3.94)
12–17 y[i]	2637	10.5 (0.78)	635	24.1 (3.22)	140	22.1 (5.97)	968	36.7 (3.97)
18–21 y[i]	1173	7.2 (0.9)	435	37.1 (5.78)	k	k	515	43.9 (7.01)

	k	% (SE)	k	% (SE)		k	% (SE)
Depression							
0-4 y[a]	k		k			k	
5-11 y[j]	404	1.4 (0.27)	120	29.6 (7.69)		208	51.6 (8.56)
12-17 y[j]	1289	5.1 (0.57)	330	25.6 (4.31)	81	492	38.1 (6.41)
18-21 y[g]	1435	8.8 (1.16)	621	43.3 (6.43)		520	36.2 (5.8)
Autism							
0-4 y[j]	40	0.2 (0.09)	k	k		k	k
5-11 y[j]	313	1.1 (0.21)	75	24.1 (7.81)		32	80.0 (14.59)
12-17 y[j]	144	0.6 (0.19)[j]	80	55.4 (16.12)		185	59.1 (9.87)
18-21 y[j]	129	0.8 (0.38)[j]	72	56.2 (24.79)[j]		65	45.3 (14.14)

[a] Denominator is all children in the sample.

[b] Denominator is children with the selected condition.

[c] Includes NVNMDS (nonvitamin, nonmineral, dietary supplements), special diets, homeopathy, biofeedback, relaxation techniques (meditation, guided imagery, progressive relaxation, and deep breathing), yoga, tai chi, qi gong, chiropractic and osteopathic manipulation, massage, movement therapies (Feldenkrais, Alexander technique, Pilates, and Trager).

[d] Denominator is children with the selected condition who used complementary therapies.

[e] Denominator is children with the selected condition who used vitamin and mineral supplements.

[f] Includes multivitamin or mineral combination, calcium, chromium, coral calcium, folic acid/folate, iron, magnesium, niacin, potassium, selenium, vitamin A, vitamin B complex, vitamin B_6, vitamin B_{12}, vitamin C, vitamin D, vitamin E, vitamin K, zinc, and vitamin packets.

[g] Question wording asked if respondent had condition, but not whether it was diagnosed by doctor or health professional.

[h] Question on anxiety asked if respondent had condition, but not whether it was doctor diagnosed; phobia or fears applies to doctor diagnosed only.

[i] Question applied only to conditions diagnosed by doctor or other health professional.

[j] Estimate has a relative standard error of greater than 30% and less than or equal to 50% and does not meet the standard of reliability or precision.

[k] Estimate has a relative standard error greater than 50% and is not shown.

evidence-based hypotheses in addition to softer clinical outcomes. Given available resources, investment in large clinical efficacy trials must be justified either by particularly promising preliminary results in smaller studies or by a compelling public health need (eg, safety information). There also remain major gaps in knowledge about both adult and pediatric safety profiles of most complementary and alternative medicine (CAM) natural products because small studies have not been sufficiently powered to precisely quantify adverse effects.

Studies of Natural Products in Pediatric Populations

Natural products (herbs, supplements, dietary manipulations, and probiotics) are the most commonly used complementary therapy, with an estimated $23 billion in total consumer expenditure in 2007.[16] Most of the claims about use of CAM natural products to treat behavioral health conditions in children are based on data from small, open-label, inadequately controlled trials or case studies; and many of them were conducted in adults. There is no single definitive large-scale trial of a natural product for these indications in children.[30] Nonetheless, many herbal medications are touted as effective treatment of anxiety, depression, ADHD, autism, and sleep disturbances. They include belladonna, cannabis, oats, chamomile, ginkgo, St. John's wort, hops, lavender, kava, American ginseng, mistletoe, valerian, omega-3 fatty acids, pycnogenol, carnitine, and probiotics,[31–34] but only a few have been rigorously studied. Furthermore, little is known about the safety or appropriate dosing of natural products in children.

Many studies in pediatric patients lack sufficient size or rigor to allow evaluation of safety or effectiveness. As a result, the evidence base for virtually all of the natural product treatments is minimal. Even when certain complementary treatments have been found to be effective, they may be not clinically useful because of their adverse effects (eg, kava seems useful for anxiety, but is hepatotoxic).[35,36] In addition, some natural products can produce significant drug-herb interactions (eg, St. John's wort), caused by their cytochrome P450 (CYP) properties.[31]

Like other complementary interventions, natural product treatments are often in widespread use despite a lack of adequate safety or efficacy information. Probiotics are used frequently in the treatment of autism on the hypothesis that children with autism may have abnormal gut flora and increased intestinal permeability. Treatment with antibiotics for presumed bowel bacterial overgrowth seems to result in only temporary changes in bowel flora, which has led to the inference that ongoing use of probiotics might be necessary to ensure normal bowel flora. Despite widespread use and anecdotal reports of efficacy, there are no well-designed studies concerning the impact of probiotics in the treatment of autism.[32] The potential risks of the use of probiotics and antibiotics in this clinical condition are not well described, although the indiscriminate use of antibiotics without clear-cut benefit is widely condemned in medicine.

An additional important consideration is the question of dosing and the impact of developmental changes on pharmacokinetics (PK) and pharmacodynamics (PD) in the pediatric population. Children are unique patient populations because they not only differ physiologically and anatomically from adults but also experience rapid changes in growth and development in the course of their childhood.[33] These developmental anatomic and physiologic changes often have major impact on the PK/PD profile for drugs and natural products, because of developmentally dynamic and variable changes in absorption, distribution, metabolism, and elimination. Our incomplete understanding of the developmental maturation of natural product disposition (PK) and effects (PD) poses a significant challenge to the development of age-appropriate dosing regimens and complicates adverse events risk assessment. However, the National Institute of Child Health and Human Development Pediatric Pharmacology

Research Unit (PPRU) Network have used population PK/PD analysis in pediatric populations, successfully identifying predictive covariates for conducting pediatric PK/PD studies. This methodology has enabled investigators to quantitatively assess the separate effects of growth and development on drug disposition in a manner not available before PPRU Network.[34]

The evidence base concerning complementary natural products treatments requiring a substantial expansion to elucidate questions regarding safety, efficacy, drug interactions, dosing protocols for youths of different ages, and clarification of indications and contraindications for treatment.

NCCAM Natural Product Integrity Policy

As a result of NCCAM's commitment to the rigorous scientific investigation of natural products used in complementary and integrative health care, studies of many natural products (eg, dietary supplements, botanicals) require rigorous and special quality control procedures, particularly in cases in which the product is not regulated by the US Food and Drug Administration (FDA) as a drug. The NCCAM Natural Product Integrity Policy provides guidance on the kinds of information required by NCCAM for different types of products before they can be used in both mechanistic and clinical research. NCCAM guidance is offered for a variety of natural products, including simple organic substances, complex botanic products, complex animal products, probiotics, refined products, and placebos. It applies to all study agents not acquired through a competitive process or developed by NCCAM-supported research-grade product development contractors or grantees.

In the context of the NCCAM Natural Product Integrity Policy, the term natural product refers to any substance of natural origin or its synthetic alternative. Product integrity refers to the entirety and completeness of information about a product that ensures it meets NCCAM policy requirements. The requested information helps provide the investigator, NCCAM, and the public with the requisite level of confidence that the research will yield definitive and reproducible results (see NCCAM Natural Product Integrity Policy: http://nccam.nih.gov/research/policies/naturalproduct.htm).[35]

POTENTIAL DRUG INTERACTIONS BETWEEN PRESCRIPTION MEDICATIONS AND NATURAL PRODUCTS

Concomitant use of complementary health products and psychotropic drugs for mental health conditions is frequent. Hence, patients who are using herbal medicines in conjunction with conventional drugs are at risk for potential drug interactions.[37] The interaction of herbal medicines with prescribed drugs presents significant safety concerns, especially for drugs with narrow therapeutic indices (eg, lithium, lamotrigine). Because the PK or PD of the drug may be altered by combination with natural products, severe and perhaps even life-threatening adverse reactions may occur in clinical practice.[36] Some of these products are known to produce significant drug-herb interactions (eg, St. John's wort) mediated by CYP,[31] but data regarding interactions of prescription pharmaceuticals with most natural products are minimal. St. John's wort has monoamine oxidase inhibitor and selective serotonin reuptake inhibitor properties, so concomitant administration of St. John's wort with these inhibitors should be avoided to prevent serotonin syndrome.[38] Furthermore, St. John's wort is a CYP 3A4 inducer, and a few case reports have suggested its inhibition of CYP1A2, so concomitant administration of St. John's wort with substrates of these pathways can be problematic.[36]

Valerian is another herbal medicine with documented interactions with psychotropic drugs. Valerian may potentiate the effects of barbiturates and other central nervous system (CNS) depressants, and a possible interaction between valerian root and fluoxetine has been reported.[39] There have been case reports of a possible interaction between ginseng and the monoamine oxidase inhibitor phenelzine, CNS stimulants, and haloperidol.[40] In addition, at least 1 case report has documented ginseng as the likely agent in a manic episode,[36] so its use in combination with drugs that potentially induce mania should be approached with caution. Ginkgo biloba extracts may lower seizure threshold in individuals with epilepsy, so gingko is contraindicated in patients taking drugs that lower seizure threshold, such as antidepressants.[40] Although drug interactions between herbal medicines and psychotropic drugs have been documented, most are case reports, and FDA reporting is not required. Therefore, the frequency of drug-herb interactions remains unknown.

NCCAM's Research Priorities for Mind and Body Approaches (Development of the Intervention)

In NCCAM's third strategic plan, one of the objectives described is to advance research on mind and body interventions, practices, and disciplines (http://nccam. nih.gov/about/plans/2011).[1] The term mind and body encompasses a diverse group of interventions, which are grouped together because they present similar challenges in designing rigorous and definitive clinical studies, such as difficulties with blinding, measurement of subjective outcomes, lack of detailed characterization or manualization, and uncertainty about underlying biological mechanism. The strategies to advance mind and body research include: harnessing state-of-the-art technologies and approaches, supporting translational research to build a solid biological foundation for future efficacy and effectiveness studies, and supporting clinical evaluation and intervention studies.

In the development of mind and body interventions, it is important to conduct preliminary studies to assess feasibility, optimize the intervention, and show a strong signal of beneficial impact. A 2-stage model has been proposed for behavioral intervention development and testing, which has applicability to mind and body interventions.[41] NCCAM has proposed a modified version of this staged approach, depicted in **Fig. 1**, for mind and body intervention research. The stepped approach for mind and

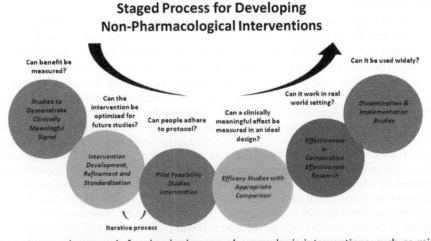

Fig. 1. A staged approach for developing nonpharmacologic interventions, such as mind and body interventions.

body research consists of the following steps: proof of concept; intervention refinement; pilot testing for feasibility and acceptability; efficacy or effectiveness studies; and dissemination/implementation studies. Often researchers and the public are most interested in whether or not a particular intervention is effective for a given condition. However, it is important to first conduct the necessary intervention refinement and pilot studies to be sure that the intervention tested in a definitive but complicated, lengthy, and expensive efficacy or effectiveness trial has been optimized for effect, feasibility, fidelity, and adherence.

The application of this staged approach to the development of mind and body interventions for pediatric and adolescent mental health conditions requires particular attention to intervention refinement and pilot testing. Researchers may need to adapt interventions to make them developmentally appropriate depending on the age and functional level of the population of children being studied. For example, studies of mindfulness meditation may not be developmentally appropriate for young children with autism, but yoga may be more suitable and has been studied in a small uncontrolled pilot trial.[42] There have been pilot studies of meditation and mindfulness-based stress reduction in adolescents,[43–45] but few if any studies on the developmental appropriateness of these mindfulness interventions in younger pediatric populations. In some situations, it may be possible to modify aspects of interventions to make them more developmentally appropriate. For example, in mindfulness-based stress reduction training, it may be necessary to discard certain elements of the intervention or to make instructions more appropriate for children. A few small RCTs of meditation have been conducted in youth with ADHD, but the small number of participants limits the ability to draw any conclusions about efficacy of meditation for ADHD.[46] If current interventions are not acceptable or feasible, additional testing of the refined intervention in an iterative process may be needed to determine whether a feasible and acceptable intervention can be developed. As an example, the Mindful Attention Awareness Scale in Adolescents is a measurement tool that has been adapted and validated in normative and psychiatric populations to assess mindfulness in adolescents.[46] Additional measurement tools may be needed or may need to be adapted for research studies in pediatric populations (eg, proxy reports by the parent or rewriting adult-based measures).

Unique challenges arise in pediatric and adolescent research regarding acceptability and adherence to study interventions. Particularly in the adolescent population, peer pressure and acceptance can create challenges for ensuring that teens adhere to treatment interventions[47] or can be harnessed in group settings to enhance adherence. Research is needed to determine if children and adolescents find it acceptable to adopt mind and body practices such as tai chi, qi gong, yoga, or other practices. The intensity of the intervention needs to be considered in the context of the child's busy schedule of school, homework, activities, and family time.

Research Methodology, Challenges, and Public Health Impact

Although all investigators who perform clinical trials face many challenges to produce quality research, those who study natural products and other complementary and alternative interventions face another level of challenges, particularly in child and adolescent populations.

Recruitment

The ability to recruit enough individuals to obtain adequate statistical power is always a key consideration to the investigator and to funding agencies. Recruitment may be affected by many factors, such as the population served, the location of the research site, and the presence of competing studies in other institutions and within the same institution.[48] Recruitment into complementary and integrative medicine trials presents several unique challenges. There may be initial public enthusiasm to try a new natural approach, but frequently people are less interested in entering trials if they may receive either placebo or a conventional treatment that they would rather avoid. Also, natural products are frequently widely available at local health food stores or pharmacies, so potential subjects can try the product on their own.

Characteristics of patients

It has been suggested that clinical trials of natural products and other complementary and integrative therapies may attract a different population compared with studies of pharmaceutical psychotropics. This supposition is difficult to assess. The authors (D.M. and M.R.) have noticed that patients who enter studies of natural products often describe a strong conviction that natural remedies are better and healthier for them than pharmaceutical drugs, whereas patients who enter studies of pharmaceutical drugs may have different biases toward specific types of treatments. Does the belief in a particular treatment increase the chances of placebo effects? A meta-analysis found no difference in placebo response rates between natural and pharmaceutical antidepressants in depression trials.[11] Similarly, in a recently published study[49] investigating of the efficacy of St. John's wort in minor depression, the placebo response rate was comparable with the response rates for either St. John's wort or the active control, citalopram. On the other hand, a recent reanalysis of the 2002 Hypericum Depression Trial Study Group study[50] suggested that patients who believed that they were receiving St. John's wort as opposed to sertraline (active control) or placebo seemed to have better outcomes, regardless of treatment received.

In pediatric populations, one might think that patient disposition toward treatments and placebo response may be less important, because it is usually the parents who decide to bring their child into a study, and young children may not understand these issues well enough to be affected. However, children are much attuned to parental expectations, even if they do not understand the facts involved, and parents are usually informants for assessing the results; their ratings on a scale are often a primary outcome measure.

Retention

Once patients are recruited into a study, it is important to retain them for the full duration, barring safety concerns that may necessitate the immediate discontinuation of treatment. Retention is a particular challenge in depression trials, which have dropout rates in the range of 20% to 30%, often caused by side effects or lack of individual improvement. Although the Freeman 2010[11] meta-analysis found no differences in overall dropout rates in CAM versus non-CAM studies, non-CAM studies had a higher dropout rate because of adverse events. However, there is a tendency toward an apparent rapid disillusionment among patients who come in to CAM studies, perhaps because of unrealistic expectations about miracle cures.[51]

Blinding

In natural products studies, patient blinding may be more of a challenge than in studies of pharmaceutical drugs. Many natural products have distinctive smells or tastes (eg, valerian), or unique side effects (eg, St. Johns' wort), which risk early patient unblinding.[51,52] Designing placebos with similar smells or tastes to the natural product under study can be complicated but is important.

Identifying an appropriate control condition for manual therapies is challenging. Individuals may have an expectancy bias that confounds response to treatment. This bias may lead to differential dropout rates that jeopardize the study and may create havoc with traditional statistical analyses. Study personnel may also introduce bias: is the practitioner able to perform the control condition in a manner that does not suggest that cit may be less effective? Rater bias or unblinding may also enter: how are personnel responsible for assessing efficacy kept masked to the treatment condition? This is a particularly vexing issue because it risks creating a Yogi Berra situation, "I would not have seen it if I had not believed it." Acupuncture is especially difficult to blind, because the treater cannot be blinded. Also, putative sham acupuncture procedures (eg, nonpenetrating needles) produce significant response rates when compared with nonacupuncture treatments,[53] or may be detected as different from real acupuncture if the patient has previous experience with acupuncture.[54] Children may be easier to blind, because they may be too young to understand the difference between active treatments and placebos and may be less concerned about what they are taking. Parents would need to be advised to not try to influence the child's belief based on their own impressions.

Individualization of treatment

Certain CAM therapies, such as homeopathy[55] and acupuncture,[56] involve individualized treatment protocols based on each patient's characteristics and symptoms. In a clinical trial, ideally all patients assigned to active therapy should receive the same intervention or at least the same decision tree, but this may seem to philosophically go against the principles underlying the particular therapy practice. Our group has recently performed 2 open studies of acupuncture for depression, using a standardized fixed acupoint protocol for all participants, with excellent results.[56,57] Controlled studies using this approach are under development.

Variability of active ingredients

A particular brand of a natural product may differ significantly from another. Different manufacturers have different methods for extracting and preparing the remedy from the herb or plant, and this may produce different proportions of active ingredients.[52] Therefore, conclusions drawn from a clinical trial of a herbal product may need to be interpreted with caution, particularly regarding dosing and toxic effects.

Regulation by the FDA

Many natural products are marketed as dietary supplements. Manufacturers of natural products may make so-called structure-function claims (eg, "supports digestive function" or "improved memory"), but they may not make claims that the product treats, prevents, or mitigates a disease or condition. In general, products being investigated for the treatment of a disorder or a specific symptom of a disorder, such as high blood pressure or depression, are regulated by the FDA as drugs, and those studies must be conducted under an Investigational New Drug Application. The FDA typically requires preclinical pharmacology and PD data, animal toxicology data, and evidence of good manufacturing standards, including assessments of product stability.

Ethical Issues

In the past decade, psychopharmacology research in pediatric populations has come under fire by many factions, both within the psychiatric field[58] and outside it. Concerns over antidepressants precipitating suicidal ideation or behavior in children and young adults[59,60] and worries about overmedicating of children with conditions such as attention-deficit disorders[61] have resulted in criticism of pediatric psychopharmacology.[62] However, natural products are generally better tolerated than conventional pharmaceutical drugs and tend to have fewer side effects.[56] Consequently, they may be more acceptable to parents of young children, as well as to older adolescents, who may feel less stigmatized if they are treated with a natural product.

SUMMARY AND FUTURE DIRECTIONS

The integration of complementary and integrative therapies with conventional practice is gaining traction for the management of mental health conditions in child and adolescent psychiatry, and this trend is largely driven by substantial caregiver interest. The integration of safe and efficacious complementary therapies with proven conventional medicine may result in better patient outcomes as assessed by symptom relief, school performance, social functioning, and family/peer relations.

We have reviewed the evidence for the prevalence of complementary and integrative health care use in child and adolescent psychiatry, specifically for clinical conditions that are difficult to manage with conventional medicine. The evidence for these therapies in child and adolescent psychiatry and health is fragmentary, but some areas of promise exist for treating difficult chronic conditions. NCCAM has just released its third strategic plan, which strongly emphasizes building the evidence base for CAM. Well-designed, adequately powered clinical trials incorporating suitable controls on key promising CAM modalities (mind and body, manipulative, natural products) for children and adolescents with mental conditions are needed. The strengthening of the evidence base for personalized, individualized decision making about using complementary therapies is a guiding principle for NCCAM's research programs, and this approach holds great promise for the future of child and adolescent psychiatric treatment.

REFERENCES

1. NCCAM. Third Strategic Plan: 2011–2015. Exploring the science of complementary and alternative medicine. 2011. Available at: http://nccam.nih.gov/about/plans/2011. Accessed January 25, 2013.
2. NCCAM. What is Complementary and Alternative Medicine? 2008. Available at: http://nccam.nih.gov/health/whatiscam/. Accessed January 25, 2013.
3. Olfson M, Marcus SC, Weissman MM, et al. National trends in the use of psychotropic medications by children. J Am Acad Child Adolesc Psychiatry 2002; 41(5):514–21.
4. Zito JM, Safer DJ, DosReis S, et al. Psychotropic practice patterns for youth: a 10-year perspective. Arch Pediatr Adolesc Med 2003;157(1):17–25.
5. Maalouf FT, Brent DA. Child and adolescent depression intervention overview: what works, for whom and how well? Child Adolesc Psychiatr Clin N Am 2012;21(2):299–312.
6. Swanson JM, Wigal TL, Volkow ND. Contrast of medical and nonmedical use of stimulant drugs, basis for the distinction, and risk of addiction: comment on Smith and Farah (2011). Psychol Bull 2011;137(5):742–8.
7. Maayan L, Correll CU. Weight gain and metabolic risks associated with antipsychotic medications in children and adolescents [review]. J Child Adolesc Psychopharmacol 2011;21(6):517–35.
8. Westover AN, Halm EA. Do prescription stimulants increase the risk of adverse cardiovascular events?: a systematic review. BMC Cardiovasc Disord 2012; 12(1):41.
9. Osher TW, Penn M, Spencer SA. Partnerships with families for family-driven systems of care. In: Stroul BA, Blau GM, editors. The systems of care

handbook: transforming mental health services for children, youth, and families. New York: Paul H. Brookes; 2008. p. 249–73.

10. Davidson RJ, Kabat-Zinn J, Schumacher J, et al. Alterations in brain and immune function produced by mindfulness meditation. Psychosom Med 2003; 65(4):564–70.

11. Wall RB. Tai Chi and mindfulness-based stress reduction in a Boston public middle school. J Pediatr Health Care 2005;19(4):230–7.

12. Freeman MP, Mischoulon D, Tedeschini E, et al. Complementary and alternative medicine for major depressive disorder: a meta-analysis of patient characteristics, placebo-response rates, and treatment outcomes relative to standard antidepressants. J Clin Psychiatry 2010;71(6):682–8.

13. Deligiannidis KM, Freeman MP. Complementary and alternative medicine for the treatment of depressive disorders in women. Psychiatr Clin North Am 2010; 33(2):441–63.

14. Reynolds WM, Coats KI. A comparison of cognitive-behavioral therapy and relaxation training for the treatment of depression in adolescents. J Consult Clin Psychol 1986;54(5):653–60.

15. Murray LL, Kim HY. A review of select alternative treatment approaches for acquired neurogenic disorders: relaxation therapy and acupuncture. Semin Speech Lang 2004;25(2):133–49.

16. Achenbach TM, McConaughy SH, Howell CT. Child/adolescent behavioral and emotional problems: implications of cross-informant correlations for situational specificity. Psychol Bull 1987;101(2):213–32.

17. Barnes PM, Bloom B, Nahin RL. Complementary and alternative medicine use among adults and children: United States, 2007. Natl Health Stat Report 2008;(12):1–23.

18. Birdee GS, Phillips RS, Davis RB, et al. Factors associated with pediatric use of complementary and alternative medicine. Pediatrics 2010;125(2):249–56.

19. Picciano MF, Dwyer JT, Radimer KL, et al. Dietary supplement use among infants, children, and adolescents in the United States, 1999-2002. Arch Pediatr Adolesc Med 2007;161(10):978–85.

20. Davis MA, West AN, Weeks WB, et al. Health behaviors and utilization among users of complementary and alternative medicine for treatment versus health promotion. Health Serv Res 2011;46(5):1402–16.

21. Bloom B, Cohen RA, Freeman G. Summary health statistics for U.S. children: National Health Interview Survey, 2010. Vital Health Stat 10 2011;(250): 1–80.

22. Centers for Disease Control and Prevention (CDC). Mental health in the United States: parental report of diagnosed autism in children aged 4-17 years–United States, 2003-2004. MMWR Morb Mortal Wkly Rep 2006;55(17):481–6.

23. Schieve LA, Gonzalez V, Boulet SL, et al. Concurrent medical conditions and health care use and needs among children with learning and behavioral developmental disabilities, National Health Interview Survey, 2006-2010. Res Dev Disabil 2012;33(2):467–76.

24. Burstein M, He JP, Kattan G, et al. Social phobia and subtypes in the national comorbidity survey-adolescent supplement: prevalence, correlates, and comorbidity. J Am Acad Child Adolesc Psychiatry 2011;50(9):870–80.

25. Eunice Kennedy Shriver National Institute of Child Health Human Development, NIH, DHHS. America's children in brief: key national indicators of well-being, 2012. Federal Interagency Forum on Child and Family Statistics. Washington, DC: US Government Printing Office; 2012.

26. Johnson EO, Roth T, Schultz L, et al. Epidemiology of DSM-IV insomnia in adolescence: lifetime prevalence, chronicity, and an emergent gender difference. Pediatrics 2006;117(2):e247–56.
27. Wong HH, Smith RG. Patterns of complementary and alternative medical therapy use in children diagnosed with autism spectrum disorders. J Autism Dev Disord 2006;36(7):901–9.
28. Hagen LE, Schneider R, Stephens D, et al. Use of complementary and alternative medicine by pediatric rheumatology patients. Arthritis Rheum 2003; 49(1):3–6.
29. Markowitz JE, Mamula P, delRosario JF, et al. Patterns of complementary and alternative medicine use in a population of pediatric patients with inflammatory bowel disease. Inflamm Bowel Dis 2004;10(5):599–605.
30. Roy-Byrne PP, Bystritsky A, Russo J, et al. Use of herbal medicine in primary care patients with mood and anxiety disorders. Psychosomatics 2005;46(2): 117–22.
31. Sarris J, Panossian A, Schweitzer I, et al. Herbal medicine for depression, anxiety and insomnia: a review of psychopharmacology and clinical evidence. Eur Neuropsychopharmacol 2011;21(12):841–60.
32. Weber W, Newmark S. Complementary and alternative medical therapies for attention-deficit/hyperactivity disorder and autism. Pediatr Clin North Am 2007;54(6):983–1006.
33. Kearns GL, Abdel-Rahman SM, Alander SW, et al. Developmental pharmacology–drug disposition, action, and therapy in infants and children. N Engl J Med 2003;349:1157–67.
34. Pediatric Pharmacology Research Unit (PPRU) Network. 1994-2010. Available at: http://www.ppru.org/. Accessed May 16, 2011.
35. NCCAM. NCCAM policy: natural product integrity. 2008. Available at: http://nccam.nih.gov/research/policies/naturalproduct.htm. Accessed January 25, 2013.
36. Chen XW, Sneed KB, Pan SY, et al. Herb-drug interactions, mechanistic and clinical considerations. Curr Drug Metab 2012;13(5):640–51.
37. Engelberg D, McCutcheon A, Wiseman S. A case of ginseng-induced mania. J Clin Psychopharmacol 2001;21(5):535–7.
38. LaFrance WC, Lauterbach EC, Coffey CE, et al. The use of herbal alternative medicines in neuropsychiatry. J Neuropsychiatry Clin Neurosci 2000;12:177–92.
39. Vickers A, Zollman C, Lee R. Herbal medicine. West J Med 2001;175:125–98.
40. Granger AS. Ginkgo biloba precipitating epileptic seizures. Age Ageing 2001; 30(6):523–5.
41. Rounsaville B, Carroll KM, Onken LS. A stage model of behavioral therapies research: getting started and moving on from stage 1. Clin Psychol Sci Pract 2001;8(2):133–42.
42. Rosenblatt LE, Gorantla S, Torres JA, et al. Relaxation response-based yoga improves functioning in young children with autism: a pilot study. J Altern Complement Med 2011;17(11):1029–35.
43. Krisanaprakornkit T, Ngamjarus C, Witoonchart C, et al. Meditation therapies for attention-deficit/hyperactivity disorder (ADHD). Cochrane Database Syst Rev 2010;(6):CD006507.
44. Biegel GM, Brown KW, Shapiro SL, et al. Mindfulness-based stress reduction for the treatment of adolescent psychiatric outpatients: a randomized clinical trial. J Consult Clin Psychol 2009;77(5):855–66.
45. Sibinga EM, Kerrigan D, Stewart M, et al. Mindfulness-based stress reduction for urban youth. J Altern Complement Med 2011;17(3):213–8.

46. Brown KW, West AM, Loverich TM, et al. Assessing adolescent mindfulness: validation of an adapted Mindful Attention Awareness Scale in adolescent normative and psychiatric populations. Psychol Assess 2011;23(4):1023–33.

47. La Greca AM, Bearman KJ, Moore H. Peer relations of youth with pediatric conditions and health risks: promoting social support and healthy lifestyles. J Dev Behav Pediatr 2002;23(4):271–80.

48. Fava M, Mischoulon D. Evaluating the data: limitations of research and quality assurance issues regarding natural remedies. In: Mischoulon D, Rosenbaum J, editors. Natural medications for psychiatric disorders: considering the alternatives. 2nd edition. Philadelphia: Lippincott Williams & Wilkins; 2008. p. 11–23.

49. Rapaport MH, Nierenberg AA, Howland R, et al. The treatment of minor depression with St. John's Wort or citalopram: failure to show benefit over placebo. J Psychiatr Res 2011;45(7):931–41.

50. Chen JA, Papakostas GI, Youn SJ, et al. Association between patients' beliefs regarding assigned treatment and clinical response: re-analysis of data from the Hypericum Depression Trial Study Group. J Clin Psychiatry 2011;72(12):1669–76.

51. Mischoulon D, Papakostas GI, Dording CM, et al. A double-blind, randomized controlled trial of ethyl-eicosapentaenoate for major depressive disorder. J Clin Psychiatry 2009;70:1634–44.

52. Mischoulon D. Update and critique of natural remedies as antidepressant treatments. Obstet Gynecol Clin North Am 2009;36:789–807.

53. Vickers AJ, Cronin AM, Maschino AC, et al, Acupuncture Trialists' Collaboration. Acupuncture for chronic pain: individual patient data meta-analysis. Arch Intern Med 2012;1–10.

54. Wu J, Yeung AS, Schnyer R, et al. Acupuncture for depression: a review of clinical applications. Can J Psychiatry 2012;57(7):397–405.

55. Bell IR, Pappas PA. Homeopathy and its applications in psychiatry. In: Mischoulon D, Rosenbaum J, editors. Natural medications for psychiatric disorders: considering the alternatives. 2nd edition. Philadelphia: Lippincott Williams & Wilkins; 2008. p. 303–20.

56. Yeung AS, Ameral BE, Chuzi SE, et al. A pilot study of acupuncture augmentation therapy in antidepressant partial and non-responders with major depressive disorder. J Affect Disord 2011;130(1–2):285–9.

57. Mischoulon D, Brill CD, Ameral VE, et al. A pilot study of acupuncture monotherapy in patients with major depressive disorder. J Affect Disord 2012;141(2–3):469–73.

58. Murray TL. The other side of psychopharmacology: a review of the literature. JMHC 2006;28(4):309–37.

59. Devi S. Antidepressant-suicide link in children questioned. Lancet 2012;379(9818):791.

60. Julious SA. Efficacy and suicidal risk for antidepressants in paediatric and adolescent patients. Stat Methods Med Res 2012. http://dx.doi.org/10.1177/0962280211432210.

61. Greenspan SI. Overcoming ADHD: helping your child become calm, engaged, and focused–without a pill. Cambridge, MA: Da Capo Lifelong Books; 2009.

62. Veracity D. Experts say antidepressant drugs cause suicides instead of preventing them. Available at: http://www.naturalnews.com/019342.html#ixzz24P56vpWO. Accessed August 23, 2012.

Index

Note: Page numbers of article titles are in **boldface** type.

Child Adolesc Psychiatric Clin N Am 22 (2013) 531–537
http://dx.doi.org/10.1016/S1056-4993(13)00048-5
1056-4993/13/$ – see front matter © 2013 Elsevier Inc. All rights reserved.

childpsych.theclinics.com

Printed and bound by CPI Group (UK) Ltd, Croydon, CR0 4YY

03/10/2024

01040441-0014